Personal Health Records
A Guide for Clinicians

To Anisa and Buthaina

Personal Health Records

A Guide for Clinicians

Mohammad Al-Ubaydli, MD
Honorary Senior Research Associate
University College London
London, UK

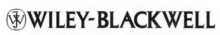

WILEY-BLACKWELL
A John Wiley & Sons, Ltd., Publication

BMJ|Books

This edition first published 2011 © 2011 by Mohammad Al-Ubaydli

Blackwell Publishing was acquired by John Wiley & Sons in February 2007. Blackwell's publishing program has been merged with Wiley's global Scientific, Technical and Medical business to form Wiley-Blackwell.

Registered office: John Wiley & Sons Ltd, The Atrium, Southern Gate, Chichester, West Sussex, PO19 8SQ, UK

Editorial offices: 9600 Garsington Road, Oxford, OX4 2DQ, UK
   The Atrium, Southern Gate, Chichester, West Sussex, PO19 8SQ, UK
   111 River Street, Hoboken, NJ 07030-5774, USA

For details of our global editorial offices, for customer services and for information about how to apply for permission to reuse the copyright material in this book please see our website at www.wiley.com/wiley-blackwell

The right of the author to be identified as the author of this work has been asserted in accordance with the UK Copyright, Designs and Patents Act 1988.

Designations used by companies to distinguish their products are often claimed as trademarks. All brand names and product names used in this book are trade names, service marks, trademarks or registered trademarks of their respective owners. The publisher is not associated with any product or vendor mentioned in this book. This publication is designed to provide accurate and authoritative information in regard to the subject matter covered. It is sold on the understanding that the publisher is not engaged in rendering professional services. If professional advice or other expert assistance is required, the services of a competent professional should be sought.

The contents of this work are intended to further general scientific research, understanding, and discussion only and are not intended and should not be relied upon as recommending or promoting a specific method, diagnosis, or treatment by physicians for any particular patient. The publisher and the author make no representations or warranties with respect to the accuracy or completeness of the contents of this work and specifically disclaim all warranties, including without limitation any implied warranties of fitness for a particular purpose. In view of ongoing research, equipment modifications, changes in governmental regulations, and the constant flow of information relating to the use of medicines, equipment, and devices, the reader is urged to review and evaluate the information provided in the package insert or instructions for each medicine, equipment, or device for, among other things, any changes in the instructions or indication of usage and for added warnings and precautions. Readers should consult with a specialist where appropriate. The fact that an organization or Website is referred to in this work as a citation and/or a potential source of further information does not mean that the author or the publisher endorses the information the organization or Website may provide or recommendations it may make. Further, readers should be aware that Internet Websites listed in this work may have changed or disappeared between when this work was written and when it is read. No warranty may be created or extended by any promotional statements for this work. Neither the publisher nor the author shall be liable for any damages arising herefrom.

Library of Congress Cataloging-in-Publication Data

Al-Ubaydli, Mohammad, 1976–
  Personal health records: a guide for clinicians / Mohammad Al-Ubaydli, MD.
      p. ; cm.
  Includes bibliographical references and index.
     ISBN 978-1-4443-3252-0 (pbk. : alk. paper)
  1. Medical records–Management.   2. Personal information management.   I. Title.
    [DNLM: 1. Forms and Records Control–methods.   2. Medical Records Systems,
Computerized–organization & administration.   3. Communication.   4. Patient Access to
Records.   5. Physician-Patient Relations. W 80]
  RA976.A4 2011
  651.5'04261–dc22

                                                                                2010049540

A catalogue record for this book is available from the British Library.

This book is published in the following electronic formats: ePDF 9781444323924; Wiley Online Library 9781444323917

Set in 9.5/12 pt Meridien by Aptara® Inc., New Delhi, India
Printed and bound in Malaysia by Vivar Printing Sdn Bhd

1   2011

Contents

About the author, vii

Acknowledgments, viii

Foreword, ix

Introduction, xii

What is a PHR?, xvii

PART 1 Your patients

Chapter 1 Sharing data with your patient, 3

Chapter 2 Protecting your patient's privacy, 13

Chapter 3 Patient communities, 19

PART 2 Your work

Chapter 4 PHRs and clinical teams, 31

Chapter 5 Educating patients, 39

Chapter 6 Saving time in your clinic, 46

PART 3 Your practice

Chapter 7 Technology, 55

Chapter 8 Law, 63

Chapter 9 Finance, 67

Chapter 10 The future, 74

PART 4 **Appendices**

Appendix A Google Health, 87

Appendix B Microsoft HealthVault, 98

Index, 113

About the author

Mohammad Al-Ubaydli, MD, is founder of Patients Know Best (www.patientsknowbest.com) and has over 15 years of experience in medical software. He trained as a physician at the University of Cambridge; worked as a staff scientist at the US National Institutes of Health; and ran the hospital chief information officer consulting practice for US hospitals at the Advisory Board Company.

Dr. Al-Ubaydli wrote six books about the use of IT in health care, including *Handheld Computers for Doctors* and *Streamlining Hospital–Patient Communication: Developing High Impact Patient Portals*. He is an honorary researcher in personal health records at University College London's Centre for Health Informatics and Multiprofessional Education, and the University of Cambridge's Addenbrooke's Hospital.

About Patients Know Best

In 2008, Dr. Al-Ubaydli founded Patients Know Best, Ltd, a personal health record company, serving clients in the United States, the UK, and Middle East. These include Great Ormond Street Hospital, the UK's largest children's hospital, Bupa, the UK's largest private health care provider, and Thalidomide Trust, providing care to all thalidomide patients in the UK.

The company has been highlighted for its innovation by several organizations, including Seedcamp, who chose them as one of the top 6 start-ups from across Europe in 2009; BusinessWeek, which named them one of the world's 25 most intriguing start-ups; and the Institution of Engineering and Technology, which highlighted the platform's innovation (Figure 1).

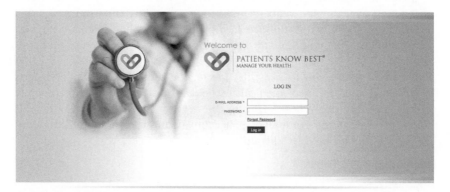

Figure 1 www.patientsknowbest.com.

Acknowledgments

My parents always taught me that if I see something that needs to be improved, I should step forward and do what I can. This is hard but my parents led by example, living a life of service to their country.

What they did not tell me, and I had to learn by myself, is that when you step forward, hundreds steps forward with you. All of them want to help and none of them expects anything in return. Some were already friends, others became friends, and all are filled with kindness.

I am grateful for the help I received from these hundreds even as space forbids me from thanking them all.

First is my mother, Buthaina, who kept my medical records as we traveled between different countries and received care from different doctors and nurses. It was she who, long before my rare genetic immune deficiency was diagnosed, spotted how prone I was to infections and boiled all water before I could drink it. Were it not for her precautions, it is unlikely that I would be alive today, and certain that I would have lost all my hearing to the ear infections of my childhood.

I am also grateful to all these clinicians that helped her and helped me. Not only did they provide the care that I needed, they cared about what I needed and they taught me how to take care of my own needs. I still remember the doctor who stabbed himself with a needle to help me overcome my needle phobia, and the nurse who patiently taught me how to inject myself as I struggled through my fears. The doctors and nurses of Addenbrooke's Hospital tolerated my childhood sulks, provided me with the independence I needed for medical school, and coached me through the risks of being a doctor on the wards.

It has been a pleasure and an honor to work with my cofounders at Patients Know Best over the past years. When I returned to England from the United States, my priority was to find the best people with whom to create the best company. Ian, Jon, and Richard: I do not know how I managed to find you, but I am so pleased that I did.

Finally, a thank you to my wife, Laura, the secret of my happiness. As a physician and author of medical textbooks, she was the first to utter the words "patients know best." During the 2 years that it took to write this book, she named our company, spelled out its mission, supported me with her salary, and brought two beautiful girls into our lives.

Mohammad Al-Ubaydli
December 2010

Foreword

Records can seem very boring. I do not think that anybody taught me anything about medical records in my 6 years at medical school. They had the status of a chair: something you used but never thought about. This was a serious omission because good medical records are fundamental to good health care. They may not be so important when tending to a man who has just lost his leg under a train, but very little medicine is that acute. Most of medicine is working with patients who have long-term conditions, often more than one. With this type of medicine, which is 99% of medicine, records are essential. Poor records are likely to mean poor care.

Unfortunately, poor records are common. I have been in hospitals about five times in my life, all different hospitals. Somewhere in the bowels of those hospitals, there will be five different records of what happened during my admissions. Quite probably, they are lost and could not be found if I were to turn up with a complication of one of my operations. I might well anyway be admitted to a different hospital, and I would either have been fixed or died by the time my records were located. Then, there will be other scattered records of when I have given blood and had the occasional diagnostic test. My general practice has an electronic record for me, but it contains almost no information and some of what it does contain is wrong. The practice may also have an extinct paper record, a small folder stuffed with letters, test results, and probably illegible accounts of consultations going back 50 years. So my medical records, like those of most of us, are fragmented, incomplete, scattered, and little use.

This does not matter too much because I do not yet have a long-term condition (or at least one I know about), but if I am run over tomorrow in Edinburgh, 400 miles from my home, and rendered unconscious, the doctors who see me will know little about me. Many patients with long-term conditions have highly complex medical histories, multiple test results, and are taking many drugs. It is essential for anybody caring for these patients (and it is likely to be several doctors, nurses, various kinds of therapists, and social workers) to be able to quickly know something about the patients, their medical history, and their current status. This can be very hard because of multiple different records and bulging, disorganized, and often inaccessible ones.

We have to do better and electronic personal health records controlled by the patient would be an important step toward doing better. Mohammad Al-Ubaydli has done an excellent job in writing this very clear book about what personal records are, what benefits they can bring, what snags must be avoided, and how they can be used practically.

On reflection, I find it very odd that we have not made much more progress toward personal health records being universal.

Why then it has not happened? As usual, I suspect that it is a combination of factors that has blocked what seems an obvious, but nevertheless, radical change. Some doctors may be resistant with worries about distressing patients and other anxieties, but increasingly doctors recognize the importance of working in partnership with patients. If they could be confident of easy access to well-organized personal health records, I think that most doctors would not stand in the way. Indeed, most will recognize that such a system could be much superior to what we have now.

Other health workers would, I think, be equally comfortable, although each group may be interested to keep its own records—so undermining the value of a single, patient-controlled record. More prosaic but ultimately more important may be the political, logistic, and cultural problems of getting the health system to build a system of personal health records. Perhaps, one of the biggest blocks has been us, the patients. We have not shown that we want a better system.

I have tried getting online access to my records. Although it is supposed to be technically easy—"simply the flick of a switch"—it took me 6 months, and neither the GP nor the practice managers were against it. When I did finally get access to my records, it was a horrible disappointment. They said almost nothing about me: only fragments of my medical history were there, and some important information was missing. I longed to be able to edit the records, add what was missing, state my values, give any possible users a sense of me. But I cannot do that. These records are about me, but they are not mine. A personal health record would be mine.

We are moving from what the American thinker Tom Ferguson called "industrial age health care" to "information age health care." This takes us from a world dominated by hospitals where doctors are authorities to a world where there is more emphasis on the ability of patients and their friends, families, and online communities to take charge of their health care. Doctors are now navigators, facilitators, and when necessary agents of action. Considerable evidence has accumulated to show that when doctors and patients take decisions together rather than taking decisions for patients then outcomes are better; patients are more satisfied, and costs are lower. Personal health records are an essential step in moving to information age health care and fostering the doctor–patient partnership.

Another step we need to take is to move from disease-based care to person-based care. Patients with multiple chronic conditions are passed from cardiologist to diabetologist to chest physician to rheumatologist with each concentrating on his or her body system and disease. The values and goals of the patient are too easily forgotten, but personal records could include statements on values and very importantly wishes of the patient that will guide the patient's inevitable death. All the time we hear the shibboleth of "patient-centered care," and surely personal health records are central to care truly becoming patient centered.

Dr. Richard Smith
Director of the UnitedHealth Chronic Disease Initiative
Honorary professor at the University of Warwick
Chair, Patients Know Best
Former editor, BMJ

Introduction

Modern medicine is wonderful. In 1799, George Washington's clinicians treated his throat infection by bleeding, and this contributed to his death (Morens 1999). In 1981 his 39th successor, President Ronald Reagan, was shot in the lung. Prompt treatment by his clinicians saved his life and allowed him 8 more years of public service and a long retirement after that.

Every year, obstetric care saves the lives of tens of thousands of mothers and children. Vaccinations have drastically reduced infant mortality all over the world. Heart attacks are no longer fatal, cancer is curable, and diabetics live for decades. When all else fails, hospices allow a dignified death.

And yet the most commonest complaint I hear from clinicians is a lack of time: they have too little time to spend with their patients, and too many patients to care for. Their frustration is because most clinicians entered health care because they wanted to help other people. They feel time-starved because they are not able to help as much as they would like to.

But the irony is that clinicians are providing more help to more patients than ever before in human history. If you are reading this book, you are one of the people making a difference.

Victims of your own success?

The problem is that you have solutions. The reason you have more patients than ever before is that you are actually able to help them more than ever before. This is wonderful news.

In the next few years, however, you will have to be even more helpful. In most societies, citizens are getting older and gaining weight, so more of them will be patients. Even those who are not sick can still become healthier with some medical attention. Those who are sick will have chronic and often multiple diseases, requiring coordination of care between multiple clinicians.

You will not have more resources. You will have more and better technology; of course, we can take that for granted for the next 10 years. But during those same years, most countries are unable to spend more money on health care than they already are. And more dangerously, we cannot count on expanding the workforce. In many countries, more nurses are retiring than are joining the profession.

So how can you continue to help more patients?

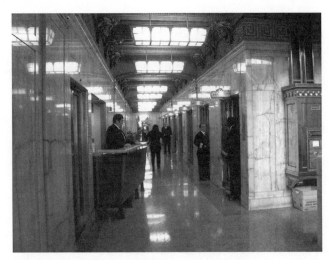

Figure 2 The lobby of the Smith Tower, Seattle, Washington, the United States. The Smith Tower is one of the last buildings in Seattle to use elevator operators rather than self-service elevators (Mabel 2008).

Ask your patient for help

Ask your patients to help you. This is the only solution that will scale. If you think about your patients as members of your team then as you gain patients and you also gain team members. The problem becomes its own solution.

It is also a really good solution. Because when a patient helps his or her clinician, they have to pay attention to their treatment. And when they pay attention, they start carrying out the instructions you know they have been ignoring in the past: they take all their medication, they exercise more, and they avoid bad habits (Mellins et al. 2000).

Every other industry has benefited from such changes. Banks are able to serve customers in more locations than ever before, 24 hours a day, because these customers use ATMs to serve themselves. Supermarkets, modern-day Cornu Copiae, offer variety, quality, and value because customers pick out their own food from the isles. But my favorite example is elevators. Think of how many elevators there are in the world, and how many people would be required if we had persisted in using an operator for each elevator.

Welcome to participatory medicine

All these changes are part of the participatory medicine movement. Yes, it is a movement, it has a website (www.participatorymedicine.org), and a journal, the *Journal of Participatory Medicine* (www.jopm.org). The traditional model is paternalistic medicine, that is, when the clinician helps the patient. In participatory medicine, the patient also helps the clinician, as patient and clinicians are part of the same team, focused on improving the patient's health. Its principles were summed up nicely by Frydman (2008):

- Patients have equal access to all data.
- Real data to make the right decisions.
- Patients are case managers of their own illnesses.
- Primary care physicians are gateways, not gatekeepers.
- Patients are coproducers of their own health.

And so this book is more about techniques than technology, and much of the discussion is about new approaches to patient care. You and your patients have to learn new habits of working together, and technology is only important because it facilitates these habits.

Davids not Goliaths

This is not a book about large organizations and their successes. There are plenty of press releases about these, and their future efforts for change will happen or otherwise regardless of the existence of this book or any other. On the other hand, large organizations are not the ones who pioneer new ways of working.

It is individual clinicians who do so. People like Ignaz Semmelweis who taught the importance of hand washing to prevent obstetric deaths; William Halstead who pioneered anesthesia in surgery; Florence Nightingale who founded the field of nursing and trained a generation of carers; and Cicely Saunders who trained as a nurse, and then a doctor, so she could found the hospice movement and provide palliative care to patients. Each of them seemed ordinary to their peers, but millions of patients benefit from their contributions every day.

And so this book talks about individuals. Large companies, such as Microsoft and Google, are included but only because their products can help individuals. National efforts, like those of the UK's National Health Service and the US Health Information Technology for Economic and Clinical Health (HITECH) Act, are also included but only because these efforts may affect yours.

Your efforts are the ones I care about the most.

How to use this book

It is important to me that you do something after reading this book. That you improve the quality of care, that you save your time, and that you enjoy working with your patients. This is what medicine is about.

I wrote it short so you can read it. Start with the first chapter. After that, read any chapter in the order you want. When you find an idea interesting, try it out. The book benefits from reading with a computer close to hand as you try out the websites mentioned.

The book itself has a website, http://book.patientsknowbest.com, which includes up-to-date materials to help you. For example, the podcast includes transcripts and recordings of interviews with personal health record (PHR) innovators highlighted in the book. The blog has news about PHRs and tips from our own company's work with clinicians and patients. And the encyclopedia provides useful information that you can share with colleagues who are getting started with PHRs. In all these pages, there are text documents you can download, audio files to listen to, and videos to watch.

And then there is me. What I enjoyed most after writing my first book, *Handheld Computers for Doctors*, is reading the messages from clinicians around the world who e-mailed me asking for advice and telling me what they had worked on. So if you get stuck, need advice, or want an introduction, make my day and send me an e-mail. My address is book@patientsknowbest.com, and I look forward to learning about your experiences with PHRs.

Patients know best

The rest of the website, www.patientsknowbest.com, is for my own company, Patients Know Best. The company provides PHR software in the United States, the UK, and Middle East. I get excited about our work and can talk about it all day. But as much as possible I have left out the company from the book. If someone else in the world does what we do, I have described their work instead of ours.

In the next edition of this book, I hope to mention your work. In the meantime, I hope you find this book useful, and that it helps you to help your patients.

Summary box

- Modern medicine is too complex for a single clinician to know everything about each patient.
- The complexity is a side effect of wonderful advances in patient care.
- The solution to complexity is to ask the patient for help.
- Participatory medicine is the new movement for patients and clinicians to work together to improve each patient's health.
- The movement can be embraced by individual clinicians like you without waiting for large health systems to catch up.
- This book will teach you how to use PHRs to support participatory medicine.

References

Frydman, G., 2008. Principles of participatory medicine. [Online] Available at: www.7word.net/?p=40 [Accessed August 13, 2008]. Mabel, J., 2008. Smith Tower

interior. [Online] Available at: http://en.wikipedia.org/wiki/File:Smith_Tower_
interior_-_lobby_02.jpg [Accessed August 6, 2010].

Mellins, R.B., Evans, D., Clark, N., Zimmerman, B., and Wiesemann, S., 2000. Developing and communicating a long-term treatment plan for asthma. *American Family Physician* 61(8):2419–2428, 2433–2434.

Morens, D., 1999. Death of a president. *New England Journal of Medicine* 341(24):1845–1849.

Acknoweldgment: Images and copyright
Part of the revolution in personal health records is the beautiful user interfaces that its pioneers are creating for patients and clinicians. I have included many screenshots in the book to demonstrate these interfaces and I am grateful to the companies and individuals who gave their permissions for all of these images.
Mohammad Al-Ubaydli January 2011

What is a PHR?

A personal health record (PHR) is a set of health records that the patient controls. This is not a new idea. In some countries, it is norm, with clinicians writing on pieces of paper that the patients carry with them to different appointments. And even in Anglo-Saxon countries, it is the norm in some specialities, for example, maternity notes in the UK.

However, there are operational difficulties with paper PHRs that have prevented mainstream adoption. For example, the patient must bring all their records with them to every visit, and the clinicians need to work with the records even the patient is not present.

Electronic PHRs do not have these problems. So we can now evaluate patient-controlled records based on their intrinsic benefits rather the operational difficulties of paper. Before we do that though, it is worth going through existing alternatives with which you may be more familiar.

Electronic health records

The idea of others controlling records in which you write is a recent one. For example, it was not until 1905 that doctors began sharing records with each other. It was the brand new Mayo Clinic that pioneered this practice as its founders recognized that providing the best medical care required a team. Each member of the team needed to see records created by every other member for the patient. And as each team member contributed their own care for the patient, they added to this set of records.

Using paper for these records had several implications. On the one hand, writing on paper is fast and easy, so it fits well with clinical workflow. On the other hand, notes are only useful to the person who reads them, not to the one who writes them. When writing, speed and brevity are essential as there are always more patients to visit and care for. But for the reader, speed means illegible handwriting and brevity means incomplete notes. This leads clinicians to ask patients questions to which the answers already exist in the notes.

Furthermore, paper is heavy so moving it is expensive, and it is just easier to keep the records in one place. But patients move and so the paper does not always follow them. The challenge is particularly acute across institutions: clinicians do not want the notes on which they rely to move to another institution when the patient receives care there. Only recently have photocopiers eased this dilemma, but photocopying is laborious and inconvenient, so complete records are rarely with the patient. All this is to say nothing of the costs of storing all the paper and the copies of the paper.

Electronic health records (EHRs) were created to solve these problems. First, computers can move and copy records almost instantly and free of charge. Second, they can index, sort, and search through these records orders of magnitude faster and better than humans can flip through paper pages. Third, text entered on a computer is always legible, and software can insist that the person writing does so comprehensively. For example, template-based histories may frustrate the person writing by forcing him or her to fill out all the information, but they delight the person reading.

Of course, there are problems. Just because information about a patient can be copied instantly and free of charge does not mean that it should be. So EHRs must include checks and balances to audit and control access. Second, the user interfaces for adding to the records must become easier so that they fit better into clinical workflow and allow clinicians to do more in less time. Speech recognition continues to improve, and the designers of templates continue to innovate. Finally, although software can search quickly, the user interfaces for starting searches must improve so that they fit closer with clinical workflow.

Ten years ago, searching the internet was hard, but then came Google and showed how easy it can be with the right technology. EHRs are not as easy to use as Google's websites are, but they get better every day.

All of which is to say that EHRs are making sharing easier. And sharing becomes more important every day as health care becomes more specialized and the care of each patient requires contributions from ever more clinicians. Sharing is no longer optional, and EHRs make it operational.

This is why in 2009 the Obama administration announced US$20 billion of funding for EHRs and why in 2002 England embarked on a £12-billion investment program. For help choosing EHR software, it is worth reading the sister book, *Finding the Right EHR: Your Guide to Electronic Health Records Success* (Gasch and Gasch 2010) at www.ehrselector.com. But the next stage in sharing is with patients.

Patient portals

A patient portal is a website that gives a patient access to the data in your EHR. The best patient portals allow interactivity so that the patient can also arrange appointments, order medications, and pay bills. In the United States, health care systems such as Kaiser Permanente (http://members. kaiserpermanente.org), the Department of Veterans Affairs (www.myhealth. va.gov), and Geisinger Health System (www.mygeisinger.org) have all improved patient care while reducing costs using patient portals. Academic medical centers such as Vanderbilt University Medical Center (www. myhealthatvanderbilt.com), MD Anderson Cancer Center (my.mdanderson. org), and the UCSF Medical Center (fetus.ucsfmedicalcenter.org) have used patient portals to help patients from across the United States. And pioneers like Hello Health (www.hellohealth.com) have transformed the patient experience by providing their EHR and patient portal to local physicians.

In the UK, Patient Access Electronic Records System (PAERS) provides family physicians with a patient portal free of charge. You can watch a video of its features, and of a patient describing the benefits they receive, at http://wiki.patientsknowbest.com/paers. Companies like 3G Doctor (www.3gdoctor.com) allow video consultations through any modern camera phone.

Patients love patient portals, so they will become increasingly common. But their spread creates a new problem: each patient has to check several patient portals to get a complete picture of their health as each health care provider sets up their own, separate, patient portal. For the patient it is better to use one website rather than several patient portals. Such a site provides all the records about the patient from all the different institutions that care for the patient. As no single institution deserves to control these records any more than another, and as data about the patient belong to the patient, it is natural that the patient should control the website.

And so we have electronic PHRs: websites with patient-controlled health records.

Personal health records

I am VERY glad my doctor still has paper records. I feel much more secure about my medical information because I know who wrote what, when and what for.

It is a comfort to me knowing that there is only ONE original of everything. Not only that, but when they leave my folder sitting on the little counter, I can peek at it and tell them about mistakes like who my current insurance carrier is and what medications I'm taking. I've found small mistakes in the past like mistakes about my weight and past surgeries.

I'd never be able to do that if my records were all digital.

Shoot Zem All (2008)

The quote above shows misconceptions about electronic records in general, and electronic PHRs in particular.

Let us begin at the end, with the primary benefit that the patient claims for paper records: that he can see the errors in his notes. This is a big benefit as finding these errors would be time-consuming for clinicians, while failing to find these errors would be dangerous for patients. With paper records, the only chance the patient gets is with the "folder sitting on the little counter." But with online PHRs, the patient can look at the notes any time they want to. They also have time to double-check with relatives, and to look up clinical terms they would not understand using the internet.

Second, electronic records in general make it much easier to "know who wrote what, when, and what for," that is, because the software automatically tracks who logged in and what they did while logged in. Paper has no such features and instead the clinicians have to manually sign at the bottom of each note. I have yet to find a nurse who will say something nice about doctors' handwriting.

Finally, it is worth discussing the "one original of everything." Even if it were true, it is not a good idea. Librarians commonly quote the LOCKSS principle: lots of copies keep stuff safe. For them, this principle is as old as the Library of Alexandria, which held so much of the ancient world's knowledge until it burned down, destroying many books of which there was only one copy. And so it is with a patient's data. Giving them an extra copy, in their PHR, creates an extra backup, which increases the safety of the data.

The rest of this book will teach you how to use PHRs and patient portals with your patients. For simplicity, I will use PHR throughout the book, except where doing something with a PHR is different from with a patient portal. But the principle is a simple one: new technology allows you to work online with your patients. And that is a good thing.

Summary box

- A PHR is a set of records that the patient controls.
- An EHR is a set of records that clinicians control to coordinate their internal team work.
- A patient portal provides patients a view of the EHR of a single institution.
- An electronic PHR allows the patient to work with their clinical team from across all institutions.
- PHRs for patients and EHRs for clinicians are complementary as each has a copy of the right data with the right tools.

References

Gasch, A. and Gasch, B., 2010. *Successfully Choosing Your EMR: 15 Crucial Decisions Records Success*. Oxford: Wiley-Blackwell.

Shoot Zem All, 2008. Comment left on medical records look good on paper. *USA Today*. Available at: http://content.usatoday.com/communities/ondeadline/index [Accessed July 12, 2009].

PART 1

Your patients

"What's next in airline self-service: customer-piloted aircraft?" An aircraft manufacturer executive overheard at after-conference drinks.

At UCL Medical School, I teach a class called "Wiki Medicine." The students have to create a wiki of medical information for patients to understand their illness. I ask them at the beginning: "if patients know more than ever before about medicine, and if patients with chronic diseases know more about their illnesses than the junior doctors you will become, what is the point of being a doctor?"

Take a moment to think about this. How are you helpful to your patients when patients can help themselves?

After a hesitant start, the students begin to raise their hands. A doctor can listen, to understand the patient's problem, and to make the patient feel understood. This doctor can examine the patient, making objective observations that help with the diagnosis. With understanding and observation, the doctor can recommend lifestyle changes, prescribe medications, or refer to colleagues. With this advice and support comes reassurance and relief for the patient. When the doctor cannot cure, they can still care, gently squeezing the patient's hand.

And as the executive at the aircraft manufacturer pointed out, passengers cannot pilot aircraft, and neither can patients carry out their surgery.

So what *has* changed because of technology? For any student who went to medical school so they could feel like the smartest person in the consulting room: the world has changed. Patients are getting a lot smarter, and they have far more time and interest than clinicians do to get smart about their own particular problems.

But for every other aspect of caring for patients, patients want their clinicians more than ever before. And as a clinician you can proceed free of the burden of needing to know more than your patient does. You can just take joy in caring about your patients as you care for them.

CHAPTER 1

Sharing data with your patient

How can we expect patients to participate in their health care if we don't give them their data?

Dr. Daniel Sands, Beth Israel Medical Centre

Dr. Amir Hannan was apprehensive about his first day as a family physician. That was because he was replacing Dr. Harold Shipman, the family physician and serial killer convicted in 2000 of murdering 15 patients in his community. The subsequent enquiry (www.the-shipman-inquiry.org.uk) concluded that Dr. Shipman had probably killed 250 patients.

The remaining patients had trust issues with Dr. Hannan.

I am still amazed by Dr. Hannan's response. Instead of backing away when he was told what surgery he would be working in, he stepped forward. Instead of ignoring the reason for his patients' distrust, he discussed it openly with them. And instead of asking the patients to trust him, he asked that they join him. You can listen to my interview with him at podcast.patientsknowbest.com (Hannan 2008).

Over the past few years, Dr. Hannan has provided his patients with access to all their medical notes through the Houghton Thornley Medical Centre's website at www.htmc.co.uk. Patients who signed up soon found what you would expect them to find: that Dr. Hannan is an honorable man, committed to the care of his patients. Hannan found that for most of his patients, knowing that he was being transparent was all they needed to know. Most of them did not register, simply choosing to benefit from his clinical expertise now that they had established a relationship of trust.

But Hannan also found out how important record access is to clinical care. He began encouraging each patient to sign up so that they could work together, as a team, to improve the patient's health.

Personal Health Records: A Guide for Clinicians, 1st edition. By Mohammad Al-Ubaydli.
Published 2011 by Blackwell Publishing Ltd.

Nobody is as smart as everybody

Across the Atlantic, Vanderbilt University Medical Center has an excellent patient portal at www.myvanderbilt.com. Dr. Jim Jirjis, a physician and VUMC's
Chief Medical Information Officer, told the story of a patient who came in
complaining of chest pain. He ordered a CT scan to check for aortic dissection
and was relieved when the radiology report showed the patient did not have
this diagnosis. A few days later, however, the patient contacted him asking
about the "lump" in the radiology report. The radiologist had mentioned this
incidental finding in the throat. Sure enough, the lump was from thyroid
cancer, and this story has a happy ending. Surgeons excised the cancer early,
and the patient has not had a recurrence.

Like Hannan, Jirjis now encourages his patients to sign up because it is
the safe thing to do. While some doctors worry that accessing the records
means that patients will discover errors and begin litigating, Jirjis and Hannan
believe that the best defense against litigation is enlisting patients' help with
finding the errors.

Safety from numbers

But what about the dangers from access? A common fear among clinicians is
what happens when patients see test results without the benefit of counseling
from their clinicians. For example, what would happen if patients found out
from a website that they are HIV positive, or if they read and misunderstood
a test result because a clinician was not there to interpret it with them?

The short answer is that in most cases, the fears are theoretical while the
benefits are tangible. But it is worth explaining why and showing a few cases
of how different clinicians picked the work flow that best suited them and
their patients.

And the first thing to say is that you do have a choice. The original reason
that test results were delivered with clinicians is that test results were printed
on pieces of paper, and the piece of paper had to go to the clinician. It was
easiest for the clinician to read out that piece of paper to the patient than to
print off another copy and send it to the patient separately. These are reasonable choices given the limitations of paper, but technology removes these
limitations. Sending out hundreds of digital copies of a test result costs the
same as sending just one copy.

So what should you choose? One extreme example is MD Anderson Cancer
Center, one of the top cancer referral centers in the world. There, all test
results are made available to the patient instantly. But that is not the extreme
part. MD Anderson is special because they were doing this from their early
days when results were printed out on paper. The results would be stored in
the paper notes, and the paper notes were stored at the foot of each patient's
bed. The patients often read the results before the clinicians came for their
ward round.

MD Anderson did this because their patients know that they have cancer. There is no harm from bad news because the patients already know the bad news and their clinicians need them to know the bad news. Everyone is on the same team fighting cancer, and everyone on that team needs to have all the information as soon as it is available.

The second thing to say is that the distress from receiving bad news without a clinician's counseling is not as bad as the distress of waiting for news until a clinician has time to counsel you. For the clinician, waiting for a result is fine because they have so many other patients to care for and because reading bad news is something they do all the day as they provide that care. But for a patient, that test result is all they can think about. And if the news can be bad, they will assume it is bad until they are told otherwise.

This is what prompted to the genitourinary medicine staff at Chelsea and Westminster Hospital to offer their SMS service. HIV is on the mind of most of their patients as they come in for testing, and the stress of waiting is terrible. Staff offered patients the choice of receiving the test results by a text message on their cell phones. Patients overwhelmingly opt into the service because it reduces the wait and because cell phones allow an intimate setting in which to read the result.

No one is told that they are HIV positive through a text message. Instead, most patients are HIV negative, and those patients are instantly told through text messages that they are fine. For the few who are sadly HIV positive, the message they receive is that they should call the clinic to arrange an appointment. A member of staff then delivers the news in person, with counseling and follow-up care. The time to diagnosis and treatment was shorter when delivering news through text messages (Menon-Johansson 2006).

The third thing to say is that your choices can be nuanced. At Vanderbilt Medical Center, the clinical team divided tests into three groups of "information toxicity." Most tests have low information toxicity, for example, hemoglobin levels of sodium concentration. Results from these tests are released immediately. High information toxicity tests include those for HIV. They are only released with a clinician's permission, and this is usually after the clinician has seen the patient. The remaining results are released after a clinician gives permission, or 2 weeks, whichever happens first. Because after 2 weeks, the benefits of clinician counseling are definitely outweighed by the patient access.

And finally, it is worth saying that most patients are more resilient than most clinicians give them credit for being. To a lay person, SOB does not instinctively mean shortness of breath. And to a patient with a psychiatric illness, reading the opinions of their clinical team can be distressing. But early experiences show that patients wait to talk to their doctor before assuming the worst about abbreviations such as SOB. And for psychiatric patients, understanding that different people have different interpretations of the same events is an important part of treatment.

But the evidence is not yet definitive, which is why the Robert Wood Johnson Foundation funded the OpenNotes Project in 2009. On the website, www.myopennotes.org, it will document the experiences of clinicians in sharing all medical notes, all the time, with patients who participate in the study. As we await the full outcomes, it is worth spelling out the benefits of sharing as most clinicians instinctively worry about the risks.

Early sharing gives your patients time to do their homework

Perhaps the strongest argument for giving patients early access to their data is that this gives them time to think about the data before they come in for an appointment. Because during the appointment, their thinking is far from perfect. There is a large body of evidence to support this view. For example, 40–80% of the medical information you provide is forgotten immediately. And the more information you provide, the lower the proportion your patient can correctly recall (McGuire 1996). Furthermore, almost half the information they remember is incorrect (Anderson et al. 1979).

But with a personal health record (PHR) at home, the patient can read all the data, look up what they mean, and prepare questions. They will make better use of their time with you.

Patients can be very good at doing their homework

Patients have incredible tools available to them. It is not just the growth in patient-friendly health care encyclopedias, but the widespread availability of tools originally designed for clinicians.

On the web, one of the earliest data points for this was membership of Medscape, a website for clinicians that had gained one million users by the turn of this century. But as early as 1996, the creators of the site had noticed that 30% of registrants were not health care professionals. For some of them it was a matter of not minding the difficulties of understanding the complex information, but for others it was about spending the time to learn to understand what their doctors and nurses already understood.

Policy makers recognize this demand. In the United States, President Bush and Congress both backed efforts to ensure that research paid for by the public would be available to the public without further payment. In the UK, the NHS Evidence website is freely available at www.evidence.nhs.uk and makes huge amounts of primary medical papers freely available. Your patients are reading primary papers.

They are even reading materials you did not think they were allowed to read. In 2009, Dr. James Heilman from Saskatchewan, Canada, posted the Rorschach test, and its answers, onto the Wikipedia. Anyone can see the ten blots (Figure 1.1) and how psychiatrists interpret patients' responses, at http://en.wikipedia.org/wiki/Rorschach_test. The posting was a controversial

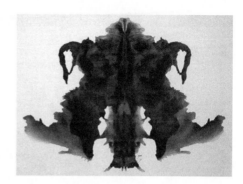

Figure 1.1 The first of the ten cards in the Rorschach test.

one, with psychiatrists and psychologists explaining that the test is not valid if a patient can read the interpretations before taking the test.

This is a shame, but it is not something you can prevent. In this case, the plates had been publicly available as far back as 1983 as part of the book *Big Secrets*, by William Poundstone. Publication in the Wikipedia simply made it easier for the public to understand the test. Clinical care that relies on keeping secrets from patients is bound to fail as the web allows easy access to these secrets.

So instead you should embrace the opportunity. And it is huge. Because just as patients now have easy access to useful data, so do you: your patients can now give you access to all the symptom diaries and home test results that can guide your care, but which were previously too laborious to collect and collate.

Patients have lots of data to share back with you

At most you have one hour with each patient each year. That leaves over 8,700 hours, which the patient spends without you. For many conditions, such as diabetes, asthma, and rheumatoid arthritis, it is difficult but important to find out what goes on during these hours. Paper diaries are common but inadequate. Filling these out is inconvenient, so they arrive to you incomplete and inaccurate. They are also out of date, and you cannot be sure whether they were filled out on the day of observation, or later on from memory.

Technology is beginning to help. This is because medical devices are increasingly digital, able to output their data streams to medical databases. The data streams are increasingly in the Continua data standard, which is compatible with an increasing number of PHRs. The details are further discussed in Chapter 7, but the point is that you can overcome many of the burdens of paper diaries.

So what data can you start collecting from your patients today?

PatientsLikeMe (Figure 1.2, www.patientslikeme.com) has demonstrated the value of symptom diaries. Thousands of patients post data in each of its

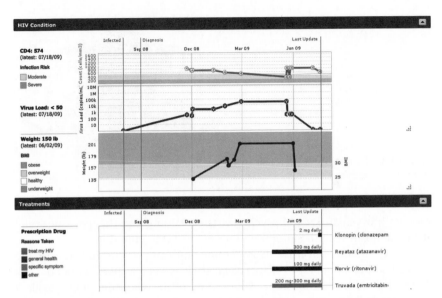

Figure 1.2 PatientsLikeMe superimposes data entered by patients about their symptoms, test results, and treatments.

patient communities. The figure above shows the clarity this brings to a patient's history and current status. Before encouraging your patient to sign up though you should explain that publishing should not mean publicizing identity. Patients should withold identifying information such as their name, address, and photograph. The next chapter discusses steps you can take to protect your patients' privacy and you can listen to the podcast interview with their director of research and development at http://podcast.patientsknowbest.com (Wicks 2009).

The nice thing about sites such as PatientsLikeMe is the printouts they provide. They are easy to understand, and each diagram shows what currently occupies several pages of handwritten notes.

But it is also possible to use PHRs to show what is impossible to explain in the notes. For example, ReliefInsite (www.reliefinsite.com) documents what the patient explains to you when they wince and grip their shoulder. Pain is complex and tactile, and while there is no substitute for examination, there is great benefit from understanding how the pain has changed in character and location. For patients, there is relief even in being understood—of finally being able to document what their pain is like and how it changes.

The website (Figure 1.3) does this through standard diagrams and templates that have been approved by pain specialists. Repeated data entry is possible through telephone voice prompts, as well as the website, for patients with too much joint pain to use the keyboard, for example. Automated time tracking means you can trust when the patient entered the observation,

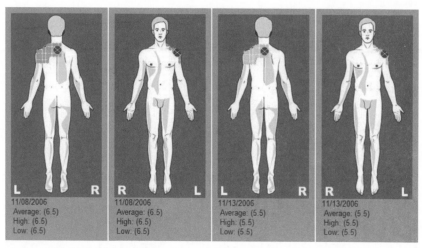

Figure 1.3 ReliefInSite visually tracks and documents pain.

rather than paper diaries where the patient may be filling out their recollections long after the event happened. And animations on the website tell the story the patient wants you to understand. You can listen to the interview with the CEO at http://podcast.patientsknowbest.com (Eberlein 2009).

Beyond documenting what happened, the patient can document what they did about it. For example, patients using ZumeLife (www.zumelife.com) enter what time they actually took their medications, what they ate, and when they exercised. Although the company started off by making dedicated devices, it now offers its software on popular devices like the iPhone. The software reminds the patient of their medication schedule. This is convenient because most patients carry a phone with them, and an increasing number of these phones include internet connectivity. As the patient enters all these data, they become available to you to on ZumeLife's website (Figure 1.4).

Patients have useful data that have not traditionally been captured

I hope that these examples have got you thinking: What else can I collect from patients? Because after technology facilitates a quantitative improvement, it becomes good enough for a qualitative improvement, a leap in capability. PHR technology allows you to collect data that have never been collected before.

The best examples of these data are the ones you will come up with. These are data items that you, your colleagues, and your patients decide that you need, and then decide to collect. If you need help, send me a message on book@patientsknowbest.com. But here are two initiatives to think about.

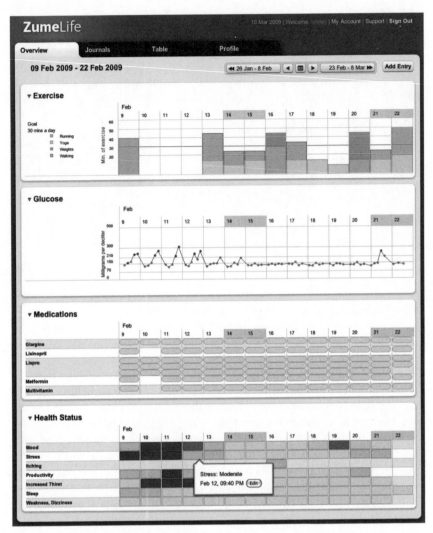

Figure 1.4 ZumeLife reminds about and tracks actions.

First is the National Institutes of Health's Patient-Reported Outcomes Measurement Information System (www.nihpromis.org). This is a set of questions that allow you to understand the patient's experience, including their physical, mental, and social health.

The questions are useful because they have been rigorously tested and validated as assessment tools. They are also modular and branching. Rather than asking the patient over scores of questions, the questions are grouped into different domains, and within each domain the questions change depending on earlier answers. For example, if the patient reports mental health symptoms, they will get detailed questions about their sleeping patterns.

In 2009, the Robert Wood Johnson Foundation captured researchers' imaginations with a US$10-million grant program called Project HealthDesign (www.projecthealthdesign.org). Its aim was to collect observations that are not recorded in traditional health records but which patients do care about. This is because traditional records revolve around data collected during, and important to, each clinical episode. But patients do not live from clinical episode to clinical episode. Observations of daily living are different but health-related information. For example, is the patient's stress high because of family or work pressures? Does their chronic pain spike with a sudden change in temperature? These data would never make it into a traditional health record, but are just as important to many people as standard clinical data are to clinicians (Project HealthDesign 2009). PHRs can help patients collect these data for you.

Shared data and shared control

Patients' contributions present a dilemma: who is in control? This dilemma is new. With paper notes, creating an extra copy is expensive, most patients are happy that their doctor is the one who should store the only copy, and possession means control.

But as soon patients have a copy of the notes, they can start making changes. In fact, you want them to do so as they correct errors and add data.

For most clinicians, this possibility is an uncomfortable one. It is important to understand that the discomfort is not from the patient's ability to make changes, but it is from your inability to know what changes the patient made.

With paper, clinicians are used to figuring out who did what, even if the process is not efficient. You know the handwriting of your colleagues. Different handwriting in the same set of notes means there is at least one amendment. You might even be able to guess the relative dates of the amendments from the appearance of the ink.

The user interface for electronic PHRs does not give you such clues, even if the tools are much more sophisticated. With our own software at Patients Know Best, we gradually switched on the ability for patients to make amendments so that clinicians could gradually learn the new clues. We also designed the user interface to clearly show which facts came from the patient, which have yet to be checked by a clinician, and which have already been double-checked.

The double-checking is not because you should not trust your patient. With most of your patients, you already believe most of what they say. Most of the errors are accidental, for example, the patient forgot or misunderstood a detail. Very rarely are the errors deliberate, with the patient actively trying to mislead clinicians. So this is not about trust. Rather, this is about letting you check what you know is important to check, so that you can trust the rest.

This trust is important if we are to achieve what most clinicians and patients instinctively feel to be the right thing to do: that there should be a unified set of records, and that everyone should add their amendments to this set. This is why PHRs are crucial in allowing patients to participate in their care.

Summary box

- Sharing data with your patients helps them trust you and help you.
- The risks of sharing data are low, and you can lower them further by gradually testing out sharing.
- Patients want access to the data you have about them.
- Giving early access to data lets patients learn more and better about their conditions.
- Patients want to learn about their conditions.
- Patients have lots of useful data to share back with you.
- Some of the most interesting data to get from patients have never been traditionally captured in medical records.
- Sharing data means sharing control and ownership, and these are worth striving for as you work with your patients to improve their health.

References

Anderson, J.L., Dodman, S., Kopelman, M., and Fleming A., 1979. Patient information recall in a rheumatology clinic. *Rheumatology Rehabilitation* 18(245):55.

Eberlein, F., 2009. Interview with Fred Eberlein from ReliefInSite. *Patients Know Best podcast*. [Online] Available at: http://podcast.patientsknowbest.com/2009/10/01/interview-with-fred-eberlein-from-reliefeinsite/ [Accessed July 27, 2010].

Hannan, A., 2008. Interview with Dr Amir Hannan. *Patients Know Best podcast*. [Online] Available at: http://podcast.patientsknowbest.com/2008/12/21/interview-with-dr-amir-hannan/ [Accessed July 27, 2010].

McGuire, L.C., 1996. Remembering what the doctor said: organization and older adults' memory for medical information. *Experimental Aging Research* 22(403):28.

Menon-Johansson, A.S., McNaught, F., Mandalia, S., and Sullivan, A.K., 2006. Texting decreases the time to treatment for genital *Chlamydia trachomatis* infection. *Sexually Transmitted Infections* 82(1):49–51.

Project HealthDesign, 2009. Rethinking the power and potential of personal health records. *Robert Wood Johnson Foundation*. [Online] Available at: http://www.projecthealthdesign.org/ media/file/E-primer_3.pdf [Accessed July 27, 2010].

Wicks, P., 2009. Interview with Dr Paul Wicks from PatientsLikeMe. *Patients Know Best podcast*. [Online] Available at: http://podcast.patientsknowbest.com/2009/08/05/interview-with-dr-paul-wicks-from-patientslikeme/ [Accessed July 27, 2010].

CHAPTER 2

Protecting your patient's privacy

Whatever I see or hear in the lives of my patients, whether in connection with my professional practice or not, which ought not to be spoken of outside, I will keep secret, as considering all such things to be private.

Hippocratic Oath, www.nlm.nih.gov/hmd/greek/greek_oath.html

Most healthcare websites have a Privacy Policy. Naturally, we do too. But at PatientsLikeMe, we're more excited about our Openness Philosophy. It may sound counterintuitive, but it's what drives our groundbreaking concept. You see, we believe sharing your healthcare experiences and outcomes is good. Why? Because when patients share real-world data, collaboration on a global scale becomes possible. New treatments become possible. Most importantly, change becomes possible. At PatientsLikeMe, we are passionate about bringing people together for a greater purpose: speeding up the pace of research and fixing a broken healthcare system.

PatientsLikeMe openness policy,
www.patientslikeme.com/about/openness

If you think storing data online is dangerous for privacy, spare a thought for Charles Gordon, Jr. His wife, Ann Chamberlain-Gordon, suspected him of infidelity. As an award-winning forensic scientist, she knew exactly what to do: sequence the genes she found in his underwear. The evidence was presented by her lawyer during the divorce proceedings (Aldhous and Reilly 2002).

Her mistake, however, was to sequence using her employer's equipment. As her employer was the state government, Gordon's lawyers made the case that this was misuse of government property; her employer agreed, and they fired her a few months later.

For US$100 at Test Infidelity (www.testinfidelity.com) she could have kept her job.

Genetic privacy is just one of the difficulties introduced by advances in medical information technology. At the time of writing, the UK's Human

Personal Health Records: A Guide for Clinicians, 1st edition. By Mohammad Al-Ubaydli.
Published 2011 by Blackwell Publishing Ltd.

Genetics Commission has taken a lead by floating for public comment a law that "non-consensual analysis of DNA would need a qualifiable consent." But around the world, there is no protection against the risks of revealing health information from the constant shedding of skin and hair with genetic materials.

PHRs help and hinder security

You must do your part to keep your patient's records secure. Security means preventing inappropriate access, but also ensuring appropriate access.

Preventing inappropriate access is harder than ever before with the internet. Computers are designed for copying data; saving copies of data costs very little; and advertising around the data generates billions of dollars per year for the likes of Google. So it is easy to accidentally divulge information, hard to reclaim it, and impossible to stop Google from permanently recording this accident.

Patients are rightly worried. In the press, attacks are usually attributed to malicious hackers. But all personal health record (PHR) systems come with rigorous security protocols for this very threat. The more problematic threat, however, is a malicious individual gaining access with you unwittingly helping. Your institution's IT security team exists to defend against such attacks. The team needs your help so follow their instructions: choose a long password, do not give out that password, and lock your computer when you are not using it.

The other scenario that makes it to the press is clinicians taking copies of data home and losing the copy. For example, on May 3, 2006, the laptop and hard drive were stolen from the home of an employee of the Department of Veterans Affairs. The laptop and external hard drive contained the names, birth dates, and social security numbers of 26.5 million current and former service members (Lee 2006).

Do not do this. Do not take the patient's data home. And if you must copy the patient's data from your work computer, encrypt it using software that your IT security team gives you.

On the other hand, ensuring appropriate access is easier with PHR systems because they provide at least one extra copy of the data to your internal one. Furthermore, PHR companies such as Google, Microsoft, and Patients Know Best are experts at making frequent, reliable backups.

PHRs allow privacy

Privacy is harder than security and less well discussed. It is the ability of the patient to say whose access counts as appropriate.

There are many threats to your patients' privacy, and many steps you can take to help protect your patients. However, this section focuses on relatives because your role is particularly important and because this threat is rarely talked about.

Without PHRs, most institutions do not handle privacy correctly. For example, any woman who calls the doctor's office of my wife can find out my wife's test results if she also knows my wife's name and date of birth. By contrast, if I call, with a male voice, staff members demand that consent is given over the phone by my wife, or at least, by a woman who knows my wife's name and date of birth. Furthermore, even after my wife gives permission, she has to continue to do so for every phone call because the staff does not have the tools to keep track of consent. PHRs are great for keeping track of consent.

And this is important because relatives pose an important privacy threat. The vast majority are, of course, well-meaning individuals and contribute immensely every day to the care and well-being of patients. But patients are often vulnerable, and relatives are close enough to patients to take advantage of the vulnerability. For example, parents can try to gain access their adolescent daughter's records to look her reproductive history, while physically disabled patients can be bullied into giving up their passwords.

There are two things you need to do to protect patients from relatives. First, only grant access to data after a patient has presented a photographic identification. You should not, for example, send the password to your patient portal through the mail as a relative can intercept it. Second, consider whether the patient is able to make the request for data independently of pressure by relatives. You should avoid giving access when relatives are able to bully the patient.

Of course, after you have cleared these two hurdles, you are left with all the relatives who are so helpful to patients. You should use them. Relatives can be more diligent than patients are in filling out symptom diaries and more proactive about contacting clinicians for preventive care. Giving them access to a patient's record—with the patient's permission—means they can more easily help the patient.

Advising your patients on how to protect their privacy

Your advice to your patients should be simple: do not publicly post personally identifying information about your health. Crucially, identifying information is available to employers and insurers. In many countries legislators are scrambling to protect patients by preventing employers and insurers from discriminating against citizens using health data. For example, the United States has GINA, the Genetic Information Nondiscrimination Act (www.genome.gov/24519851).

However, these laws are difficult to enforce and a lot of money is at stake. For example, in 2005, Wal-Mart Watch highlighted the measures taken by Wal-Mart to identify and discriminate against employees with high health care costs (Barbaro 2005). Furthermore, technology will only improve in the ability to index and interpret publicly available identifying information.

Conversely, it is not necessary to provide identifying information to gain the benefits of sharing publicly. For example, to get advice from others, a patient can post symptoms and photographs of any skin lesions that do not include the face. Divulging addresses, names of employers, and mobile phone numbers is not necessary. Nor should patients use a work e-mail address, or an e-mail address that includes their name (e.g., moham-mad.alubaydli@gmail.com). Simple precautions can go a long way to reducing risks.

None of which is to say that patients will follow this advice. A great example of this is the HIV group of the website PatientsLikeMe (www.patientslikeme.com) where several thousand patients post information about their HIV medical history. Photographs, location, HIV status, and all sorts of other information are posted online by these patients.

These patients believe, for the most part accurately, that they can get better care by sharing their data more widely to allow comparisons with other patients and feedback from other members of the community. PatientsLikeMe certainly makes an important contribution to the health care of these patients. But none of these benefits require divulging private information.

Of course, after you have protected patients' privacy, and advised them how to protect themselves, you still have to protect your own privacy.

Protecting your own privacy

I now live in Dover, where I work for the NHS, bullshitting for a living, no change there then

>   Comment on the social network profile of Eastern and Coastal Kent
>   PCT assistant director of strategic partnerships, Caroline Davis.

It seems to me that if you or I must choose between two courses of thought or action, we should remember our dying and try so to live that our death brings no pleasure on the world

>   John Steinbeck

You should be aware that your own data are available on the internet and you should assume that patients and journalists will access these data. This is not just the obvious and appropriate data like your medical license registration, or the office hours of the institution that you work in. Rather, it is the sites that feel like they are private but are actually widely accessible. For example, we know about the comment by Ms Davis above because it was published in the press, and we know that her employer had to take disciplinary action following the press attention. In 2009, the British press had looked at the Facebook account of the wife of Sir John Sawers, the future head of the British Secret Intelligence Service. They found out the London apartment used by the couple and the whereabouts of their three grown-up children, and of Sir John's parents.

Social networking websites like Facebook (www.facebook.com) are misleading in that they encourage a mental model of privacy but have a business model of publicity. In other words, people are comfortable sharing information because they have the impression of private conversations with friends, but fundamentally sites like Facebook benefit from spreading your messages as far and wide as possible. The comfort you should feel in Facebook is the same you should feel while in your car: it feels private, but everyone can see you.

Nor should you feel more comfortable in sites created specifically for professionals. For example, Sermo (www.sermo.com) in the United States and Doctors.net in the UK (www.doctors.net.uk) are designed for doctors and check the medical licensing data of each user before granting access. However, journalists still get access, doctors may have their accounts hacked, and even your colleagues may publicly attribute to you something you said on the private forums.

So you should assume that everything you say can be publicly shared, forever. On the one hand, this seems unfair, and it is if you think of the responsibility you have to bear compared to that of nonprofessionals. On the other hand, the privilege of being a professional is far more significant than anything a free website can offer you.

Nor is it a bad idea to act like a professional at all times. Online, think of the words of Steinbeck before you add your own. His are words to live by.

Summary box

- Advances in medical and computer technology make maintaining privacy increasingly difficult.
- You must do your part to help protect your patients' data.
- Security is preventing inappropriate access and ensuring appropriate access, while privacy is about the individual indicating which access counts as appropriate.
- PHRs facilitate privacy by putting control in the patient's hands.
- PHRs automatically track changes in a patient's consent over time so you do not need to constantly and manually check.
- Advise your patients not to publicly post identifying clinical data, even though they may choose to ignore this advice.
- Do not forget to also protect your own privacy, especially as personal opinions can be linked back to your professional status.

References

Aldhous, P. and Reilly, M., 2002. Special investigation: who's testing your DNA? *New Scientist*, Issue 2692 [Online]. Available at: http://www.newscientist.com/article/mg20126924.100-special-investigation-who-is-testing-your-dna.html?full=true [Accessed September 3, 2009].

Barbaro, M., 2005. Wal-Mart memo suggests ways to cut employee benefit costs. *The New York Times*, October 26. [Online] Available at: http://www.nytimes.com/2005/10/26/business/26walmart.ready.html [Accessed July 27, 2010].

Lee, C., 2006. Stolen VA laptop and hard drive recovered. *The Washington Post*, June 30. [Online] Available at: http://www.washingtonpost.com/wp-dyn/content/article/2006/06/29/AR2006062900352.html [Accessed July 27, 2010].

CHAPTER 3
Patient communities

[Burmese king Nandabayin in 1599] laughed to death when informed, by a visiting Italian merchant, that Venice was a free state without a king.

Schott (2002)

Technically, personal health records (PHRs) must be separate from patient communities. This is because a PHR is a patient's private set of records, while a community is a public discussion. However, the value of the data in a PHR increases greatly if a patient can learn from a community how to interpret the data inside it. Furthermore, patient communities are great examples of participatory medicine because the patients considerably outnumber the clinicians and their opinions often count as much as those of the clinicians. Finally, these communities can also be useful to you clinically, financially, and academically.

My first experience of the internet taught me an incredible lesson about the power of its communities. It was 1994, I had just spent my first month at university, and my computer science professor could not tell me how to find a particular software program I was interested in. "Why don't you go on the internet," he suggested?

Off I went to the computer laboratory and I started reading about how to use forums. Although web browsers were around in 1994, I was not aware of this, and instead struggled with black and white screens and keyboard commands. I am embarrassed to think of what I must have sounded like to the participants of the artificial intelligence forum on which I posted my question, but for some reason one of them responded by asking me what my mailing address is. I was also not aware of the dangers of talking to strangers, so I gave him my home address.

The following week, a floppy disk arrived from a Canadian university professor. The disk contained the software I had asked for.

To this day, I have no idea why he did this. He was a highly accomplished academic, and I was clearly a naive student, but he took the time to help me out. Over the past 15 years, I have learned that the internet is full of helpful people.

Personal Health Records: A Guide for Clinicians, 1st edition. By Mohammad Al-Ubaydli.
Published 2011 by Blackwell Publishing Ltd.

The power of the internet is not in the percentage of its users who are good. Rather, it is in its ability to concentrate their good actions and weed out bad ones. This is why when you search on Google, the first three results are so useful. The remaining billions are of variable quality, and the average quality is almost certainly low. But Google highlights the best in a billion, and these are very high-quality results. And in health care, the single website that comes up most often is the Wikipedia, an encyclopedia with 13 million articles built by a community of volunteers from around the world. They are called Wikipedians, and there are over 10 million registered accounts through which they edit the Wikipedia, while an unknown number of them also edit the site.

Wikipedia: the world's largest community

If you are like most doctors and nurses, the idea of anonymous volunteers writing medical information that patients then act on is one that horrifies you. And if you think your expertise is ignored when your patients learn from these volunteers, just think how dispiriting this must be to the scientists of the National Institutes of Health (NIH). Each of them is a world expert in their field and yet on a Wikipedia page any changes they make take no more precedence than those of any member of the public.

But on July 16, the National Institutes of Health ran a Wikipedia Academy for its scientists. Its aim was to teach the scientists how to participate in the world's largest encyclopedia. You can see full details at http://wiki.patientsknowbest.com/Wikipedia, but if there is one thing I can teach you it is this: if you see an error on Wikipedia, fix it.

Not that the Wikipedia has many errors. In 2005, the journal *Nature* peer-reviewed 50 randomly selected scientific articles from the Wikipedia and compared these with the same articles in the Encyclopedia Britannica. For each encyclopedia, there were four serious errors. There were also factual errors, omissions, and misleading statements in both: 162 in Wikipedia and 123 in Britannica. The difference between the two is *not* that Wikipedia has a free price, which makes its errors tolerable.

The really important difference is how the two institutions respond to errors. Britannica spent its money on a full-page advertisement in the New York Times the following day trumpeting its superiority. The Wikipedians spent their time fixing the errors. By the next day, the Wikipedia no longer had the errors identified by *Nature*, but Britannica still did. The Wikipedians even created a separate page on the Wikipedia in which they listed and fixed the errors of Britannica (Wikipedia 2005).

Fixing errors is easy. Figure 3.1 shows a screenshot of the page about influenza (http://en.wikipedia.org/wiki/Influenza). At the top of the page, there is a button labeled "edit this page." You will see a page like the one in Figure 3.2.

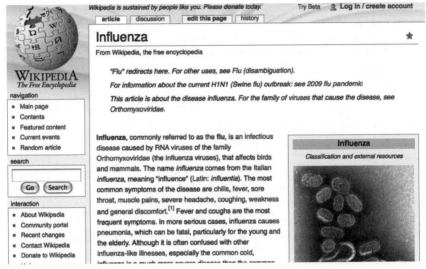

Figure 3.1 The Wikipedia page about influenza.

The white rectangle with text inside it is what you edit. Find the line which is incorrect, fix it, and click the "save page" button. Your change is now instantly available to all Wikipedia readers. In May, 6.3 million of them had accessed this page so the impact of your fix is large.

Most people are shocked when this process is explained to them. A few are so shocked that they do not believe it. If you are one of them, spend a minute

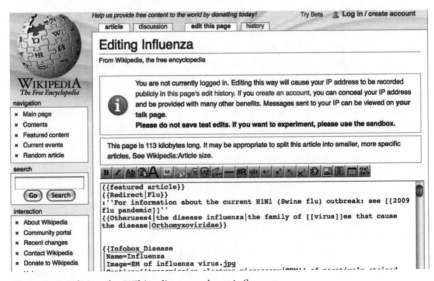

Figure 3.2 Editing the Wikipedia page about influenza.

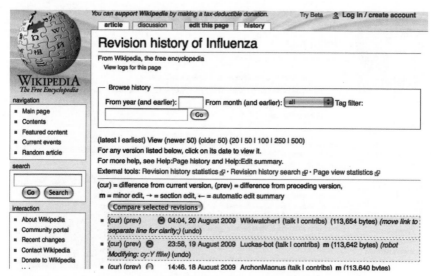

Figure 3.3 Editing history of the Wikipedia page about influenza.

trying this yourself. It is really that easy to make a change to the web's fourth most popular website, and the world's most used encyclopedia.

But for all the risks that you are imagining, the Wikipedia community produces high-quality content with a low error rate. They can do this because they have peer review tools on a scale unimaginable to the medical publishing industry. First, to the right of every "edit this page" button is another labeled "history." Clicking this for the influenza page shows the view in Figure 3.3.

It shows each change, the size of the change, and who made the change. You can select two versions and compare them to understand exactly what changed as the software highlights deletions and insertions in bright red. With a couple of clicks, you can revert to any older version. Although it appears easy to vandalize the Wikipedia, it is even easier to revert to the version that was not vandalized.

The monitoring and reversions are fast and frequent because of the commitment of Wikipedians to their site. If they see blatant damage, for example, someone completely deleting the text of an article, they quickly revert to the earlier version. But otherwise they check each change to see if it is supported by evidence. If it lacks evidence, they either try and find a citation, or they revert to the earlier version. This is exactly the process that every peer-reviewed medical publication aspires to, but none of them have 10 million passionate volunteers, and few of them use the powerful change tracking software that powers the Wikipedia.

Finally, the deliberations of these volunteers are available for you to learn from and contribute to. Click on the "discussion" button to see the ongoing discussion about the influenza page (Figure 3.4). For example, at the time of

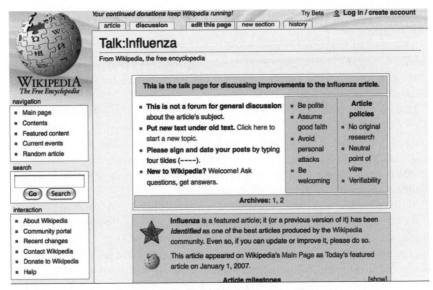

Figure 3.4 Editing discussion of the Wikipedia page about influenza.

writing, Wikipedians were discussing the importance of fever to combating pathogens; making the layout of the article less like that of a textbook; facts of the 1989–1990 flu epidemic; and the etymology of the word influenza.

For most clinicians, contributing to the Wikipedia is not a concern. A few do it because it is enjoyable, a hobby that contributes to the welfare of so many patients. Others should do so as they are world experts on a disease, something that NIH's Wikipedia Academy tried to encourage. But all clinicians should familiarize themselves with its tools of peer-review as they are so useful to understanding how to discuss clinical information with nonclinical professionals. Because such discussion is vital.

The value of communities

At least one person in your clinical team must get involved in the discussions of online patient communities. These communities provide relevancy, efficiency, empathy, and publicity.

David de Bronkart (http://patientdave.blogspot.com) shows the importance of online discussions to provide relevant information. His initial diagnosis of cancer carried a median survival time of 24 weeks. This is sobering news for anyone to hear. David is grateful for what his physician, Dr. Daniel Sands, did next: "he prescribed ACOR". Through the Association of Cancer Online Resources (www.acor.org), he discussed his case online with patients and clinicians. And there he learned what median means. Although the 50% of patients with his condition live fewer than 24 weeks, the other 50% live far longer. Fortunately, he is one of these patients, and several years on, he is still cancer free.

The median is just one example of tailored advice that patients like David need every day. Making more reference information available is not the answer as it discusses the average. But neither is there time for you, personally, to sit down with each patient.

Online discussions are efficient. When patients and clinicians teach David about the median, everyone else learns as well. The whole community pitches in to provide these answers, reducing the workload on individual clinicians as patients do far more work than we have clinicians for. And you get to learn from expert patients in conversations that would never fit into the tight deadlines of clinical appointments.

With empathy, you can also learn from patients what you are doing wrong. For example, David wrote in his blog about calling a radiology department to book an appointment (de Bronkart 2009). He was told that he did not need an appointment, and that he could just come in any time that he wanted to. So he did. And found a line with a wait that was longer than 45 minutes. He left and called to ask for an appointment but was told that it was too late for an appointment that day, but that he could book another for the following day.

The great thing is what happened next. Someone from the department read about the incident, and got in touch with him. The radiology team is now more clear about the instructions they give over the phone so that patients do not waste their time as David did.

Not only can you learn what you are doing wrong, you can learn what others are doing right. Patients discussing their care online will tell you things you colleagues at other institutions will never share with you, and continuing medical education lectures will never impart to you. For example, at the end of one appointment with a physician, I mentioned what a previous physician had done. The doctor was instantly interested and asked lots of questions. I knew that the two clinics were competing and so such information was useful as each tried to improve its protocols. When I went home, I checked the online forums for my illness. Within an hour I had information from past patients' discussions about all other clinics in the same city as my doctor.

I am not suggesting that you should spy on your competitors. I am imploring you to. Please, learn from them. Variation in clinical practice is only useful if we are trying to discover what practice works best. But arbitrary variation, because clinicians are ignorant of other practices and their outcomes, wastes medical resources and harms patients.

Finally, the publicity you get from helping patients online is better and cheaper than paying for advertising. A profile that shows the discussions you joined in and expertise you have should serve you better than advertising would.

So how do you get started?

Communicating in communities

In the beginning, it is probably best to join an existing community. Software to create your own community is relatively easy and cheap to set up. But getting patients to join your community, when they already get so much value from existing communities, is hard and expensive.

Sites such as MedHelp (www.medhelp.org) provide hosted clinical discussions. Alternatively, if you contact the patient charities for the diseases that you treat, they can provide you with a list of existing communities.

When you join a community, begin by following existing discussions. Watch how others respond for a couple of weeks before you provide your own responses. When you start answering questions, make sure you include links to pages that have further information. Avoid abbreviations, but be brief. You should include your full name and your institution's contact details so that patients can book appointments at your clinic. But having identified yourself you have an added responsibility to make sure that your comments make your institution look good. Always speak positively, focus on solving the patient's problem, and never criticize others who try and help, even if you disagree with their suggestions. Instead, focus on constructively explaining the reasons for your disagreement.

If you really do want to start your own community, you will need the help of someone technical to set up the software. The technical set-up should be fast. Open source software such as phpBB (www.phpbb.com) and putting it on your website should cost you less than US$100 per year.

But it is crucial that at least one person in your team knows how to manage communities. The Moderator Community (www.themoderatorcommunity.com) is a good place to learn the skills necessary, with documentation and mentoring available free of charge. The interview with its founder, Maria Sipka, is well worth listening to as she discusses different kinds of communities (Sipka 2009).

Finally, the same person that you would choose to manage your community can also monitor other communities for what patients say about your team. In the UK, companies such as Patient Opinion (Figure 3.5, www.patientopinion.org.uk) and iWantGreatCare (www.iwantgreatcare.org) provide tools for constantly surveying patients for their opinions and integrating this feedback into dashboards that everyone in the clinical team can look at and learn from.

More broadly, Google, Twitter, blogs, forums, and all kinds of other social media will contain comments about your team. Perhaps the easiest thing you can do to monitor them is to set up an alert with the name of your institution at Google Alerts (www.google.com/alerts). But whatever tools you use, the point is to use these tools. Communities that include patients are great resources, and you should make full use of them.

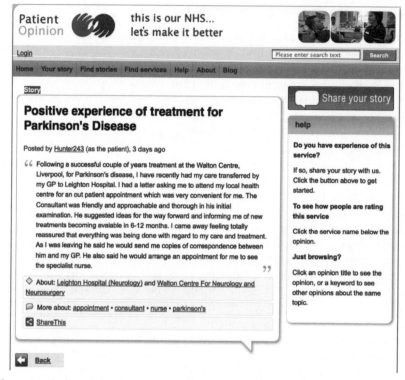

Figure 3.5 Patient Opinion monitors other communities for what patients say about your team.

Summary box

- Patient communities are complementary to PHRs because they allow the patient to learn from peers and professionals how to understand his or her private data.
- Patient communities also provide free labor to support your teaching, and can help you clinically, financially, and academically.
- The Wikipedia is the world's largest and most highly used medical resource, and it is built by a community of volunteers.
- NIH and others have recognized the value of contributing to the Wikipedia, and doing so helps you understand how to work in communities online.
- At least one person in your team should join patient communities, both to represent you and to bring teachings back to the team.
- Start by joining an existing community, and use existing community platforms, before you attempt building your own.
- Monitor what is said about you in communities so that you can improve your patient care.

References

de Bronkart, D., 2009. Customer service in healthcare (not): an all-too-true-story. *The New Life of e-Patient Dave*. [Online] Available at: http://patientdave.blogspot.com/ 2009/07/customer-service-in-healthcare-not-all.html [Accessed August 30, 2009].

Schott, B., 2002. *Schott's Original Miscellany*, 1st ed. London, UK: Bloomsbury.

Sipka, M., 2009. Interview with Maria Sipka from Linqia. *Patients Know Best podcast*. [Online] Available at: http://podcast.patientsknowbest.com/2009/09/15/interview-with-maria-sipka-from-linqia/ [Accessed August 24, 2009].

Wikipedia, 2005. External peer review. [Online] (Updated December 22, 2005) Available at: http://en.wikipedia.org/wiki/Wikipedia:External_peer_review#Nature_ .28December_2005.29 [Accessed August 24, 2009].

PART 2
Your work

CHAPTER 4
PHRs and clinical teams

Technology is nothing without technique, and new technologies need new techniques. But it takes time to invent new technologies, and still more time for the new techniques.

For example, early radio presenters simply read books on the radio. It took a while for radio formats such as plays and quiz shows to appear. Early television shows were radio ones with a television camera pointed at the actors as they read into a microphone. It took a while for television shows with actors moving and scenes changing. Early internet video sites tried to broadcast television shows. But YouTube's slogan is "broadcast yourself," and it showed the value of the internet in allowing anyone to create videos and share them with others.

And so it is with personal health records (PHRs). The technology is powerful, but you must learn new ways of communicating with your team to deliver the full benefits to you and your patients.

Everyone has to be on board

All collaboration tools suffer from the same problem: the person who does the work is not the one who benefits. Clinicians often mistakenly think that the problem is the use of new technology. It is not. For example, a doctor writing a prescription by hand must spend more time on clear handwriting and avoiding abbreviations. This does not help the doctor because they already know what they intended to write. Rather, it helps the next person along in the prescription chain: the pharmacist or the nurse who dispenses the medication. If the handwriting is not clear, or the abbreviations are ambiguous, the pharmacist or nurse must spend time figuring out what the doctor had meant. This is often much more time than the doctor had saved by writing quickly.

Medical software sometimes forces this issue. For example, prescription software often takes longer to fill out because unlike a piece of paper a computer does not tolerate incomplete or ambiguous data. It forces the doctor to spell out everything. While pharmacists and nurses rejoice, the doctor rues the day they agreed to use computer software.

Everyone in your team must understand this conflict of collaboration before they begin. If they do not, they will blame PHRs for losses in their

Personal Health Records: A Guide for Clinicians, 1st edition. By Mohammad Al-Ubaydli.
Published 2011 by Blackwell Publishing Ltd.

productivity because they are not aware of the increases in the productivity of others. Of course, if you write clearly today in the notes, you may end up benefiting in one month's time as you look again at what you wrote. But fundamentally, you must accept the sacrifice so that your colleagues and patients benefit, and teach them to make the same sacrifices so that you benefit. You will only succeed as a team if you all understand this.

Which is why it is worth starting as a small team. For example, if your institution has ten departments, each with ten employees, it is far better to have the ten employees in one department using PHR software than to have one employee in each of the ten departments do so. The lone employee in each team will likely be an enthusiast, but without the support of their colleagues enthusiasm turns to burnout and then to abandonment. That is because the person spending the extra time to benefit their team receives no offsetting benefits if the rest of the team is not spending the extra time as well. By contrast, small teams whose members commit to working together sustainably reap the benefits of cooperation and instill confidence in other teams to make the leap as well.

Train your team

Your colleagues have too much to learn and too little time to learn it in. There are three things they absolutely must make time to learn though.

First is the strategic importance of PHRs for the team. This is not something you can tell them to accept, instead you must put forward the idea in a team meeting and let your colleagues discuss it. Everyone goes through the same questions as they begin to understand the implications. Will this be dangerous to patients? Will this take up more time? Will this cause confusion? Will patients struggle to use computers?

The answer to all these questions is "no." But you have to give your colleagues the chance to ask these questions before you can begin; otherwise, they will ask the questions after you begin. If you force them to the latter, the answers will become "yes" as your colleagues hide information from the notes, which is dangerous; spend more time duplicating notes, which is unsustainable; cause confusion from the multiple overlapping workflows, which is frustrating; and fail to help the patients get passwords and use the software, which renders all this work pointless.

So give them time. What may be obvious to you after reading this book is not so to most people.

On the other hand, I am constantly amazed at how often individuals soothe each other's worries. The nurse who is worried about dangers to patients will be the one who volunteers that he spent so much time doing work that his patients would gladly do if only they were allowed to. The doctor who is worried about her own confusion will admit that most of her patients already use the internet and would, with their family members' help, cope admirably. Wait through this process.

The second training is the changes to workflow. At http://wiki. patientsknowbest.com/Clinical_training, you can watch a short video lecture I gave at the Royal Society of Medicine that teaches clinicians how to work with patients online. Send the links to the lecture to your colleagues so that they can watch it at their convenience, but you should have a group meeting in which you all discuss the implications for your work. Again, this is part of giving your colleagues time to accept and adopt.

Only then should you begin the third part of training, which is how to use the software. Start with small teams rather than large deployments, and there is no replacement for one-on-one training. Long PowerPoint lectures do not work; instead, the experienced need to sit down with the less experienced. The rest of this chapter is about this training.

Stick to patients you know

PHRs are safest and swiftest with patients your team already knows. Your notes have more information about these patients. They already have a relationship of trust with your team, and if you have personally had consultations with them in the past, you probably have a better understanding of how to interpret their writing.

It is possible to work with new patients. For example, services such as 3G Doctor (www.3gdoctor.com) provide the patient with a detailed online form that has been tested for providing a history that is close to complete. The interview with its founder is available on the podcast website (Doherty 2008).

But the service is primarily designed for patients who want a second opinion from a specialist. These patients are motivated enough to type up their entire history, and there is not the urgency of a recent injury or chronic disease exacerbation. Furthermore, the doctor follows up with a video telephone call with the patient, during which the doctor can pick up information from watching the patient speak, or seeing the affected part of their body. By contrast, most PHRs are set up for messages to go back and forth over time, and few have video features. So for the moment, within this medium, you should protect yourself and your patients.

The best way to do this is to begin with a low threshold for asking the patient to come in. If the examination would reveal something that would change your management, ask the patient to come in to see you. And if a test result would do the same, ask the patient to go to their local laboratory to get the test. As you become more comfortable with the technology, you can raise your thresholds and reduce your patients' travel. But the foundation of all of this is patients with whom your team already has a relationship.

Assume your writing is read

With all your patients, you must assume that what you write is being read always. Even if you do not think it is, for example, if you have decided you do not want to work with patients online, your writing can still be read by patients at any time. This is because the data ownership laws allow patients to request their data any time and the number of requests is only going to increase. So you need to write in a way that is patient-friendly, something medical schools do not teach very well.

Not that patients expect you to be friendly. For the most part, even when they are upset by what they read, they are still glad they got to read it. But it is helpful to you and the patient if you write objectively, especially when the news is bad. For example, if you believe the patient is drinking more than he or she is letting on you do not have to say they are lying, but you can objectively say that the liver test results are the same as those of people who drink a lot. Nor should you consider hiding your notes, or keeping a separate set of notes. Your duties as a doctor include the maintenance of complete notes and the provision of these notes as part of delivering safe high-quality care.

The one exception is for maintaining confidentiality. For example, if some-one tells you something about the patient in confidence, you are duty-bound to maintain the confidence entrusted in you. In that case, you should have a separate set of notes, and I recommend paper. The aim is to make these notes difficult to access because you are actively trying to prevent sharing. The analogy is the genitourinary medicine department in many hospitals which maintains a separate record system to maintain confidentiality, which in turn is part of good care.

But for everything else, you have to write in the notes, you have to write assuming that your patients will read it, and you have easy ways of doing so.

Finally, a note on abbreviations. In general, it is better to minimize these. Some of them are to be avoided altogether. For example, when I was training, some junior doctors considered FLK (funny-looking kid) to be clinically use-ful, and NFN (normal for Norfolk) to be funny. You know your local equiva-lents, and you should avoid them.

You do not need to avoid SOB just to avoid offending patients who misun-derstood you. They will ask you, or Google, what you meant and will arrive at shortness of breath before they wrongly assume you had meant the more colloquial and offensive SOB.

Rather, you should avoid abbreviations because they are ambiguous. The ambiguity is confusing to your colleagues, and even to you, after the passage of time. On the other hand, some abbreviations are really well established, and of course using abbreviations saves your time. You will have to find the right balance for you and your team.

Say sorry and thank you (early and often)

As your patients start reading, you should expect them to discover a large number of errors. This is wonderful. Because the only thing worse than spending time fixing errors is spending time acting on erroneous information:

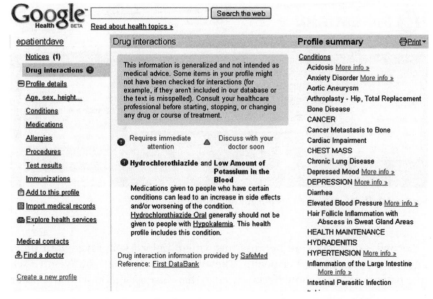

Figure 4.1 The medical records of e-Patient Dave stored on Google Health.

ordering tests, writing prescriptions, and getting referrals. All these things cost time and money and may be dangerous for the patient if the information you are acting on is wrong because your notes are full of errors.

A notorious example is the errors that Dave deBronkart found in his PHR records from Beth Israel Deaconess Medical Center (Figure 4.1). He published these errors on his blog in April 2009 (e-Patient Dave 2009), and his readers were amazed at the number and magnitude of errors. Shortly after this, Beth Israel temporarily halted its efforts with Google Health. This example is extreme because the data he received were actually from the insurance billing codes and clinicians change these to qualify their patients for free treatment. But plenty of errors were administrative, or from old diagnoses that incorrectly still appear as current problems.

You will probably find an error rate around 30%. They will not all be severe errors, but there will be errors, and it is useful to you when your patient finds them for you.

The key is how you react. First, say sorry. Do not bother going into whose fault it was. It is most likely not yours, but rather that of the hundreds of other clinicians working with you to care for your patients. Furthermore, your patient does not care whose fault it is, nor do they want the person whose fault it is to be punished. What they do want though is a clinician to take the error seriously and to care about fixing it. If the fix is fast, fix it now. Alternatively, you can ask your administrative staff to fix the more laborious mistakes. But the key is to quickly say sorry and find a way to fix the error.

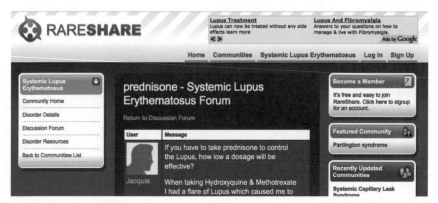

Figure 4.2 RareShare provides forums about rare diseases.

Second, say thank you. Because this patient helped you, saved your time, and cares about his or her health. They demonstrate what you want to see in a patient and you should acknowledge that, just as you do with any other member of your team.

Learn from patients

Patients can teach you much more than where the errors are in the notes. This is not to say that patients know more than you do about medicine. But individual patients do have access to facts that you do not, including side effects of medications and how they adjust their lives around these side effects. And in aggregate, patients can create knowledge about an illness that even specialists did not know. This is why you find world-class researchers on websites such as RareShare (www.rareshare.org), which provides forums about rare diseases (Figure 4.2). The specialists learn from these patients as well as teach them.

Most doctors will be too busy to use these forums, especially family physicians with so many diseases to look after. But for a practice specialist nurse, this is an excellent use of time as he or she already has to increase their knowledge within one disease group. Ask the specialist nurse in your team to spend time on forums and then teach what he or she learned to the everyone else. I promise you an eye-opening education.

Relatives are part of your team

Just as valuable as patients are their relatives. They have traditionally been kept out of the loop because of the difficulties of complying with privacy laws, and the chapter on protecting your patient's privacy has more details. But PHRs make it easy to document a patient's consent, easing your legal burden, and easy for the patient to revoke consent, easing your patient's fears. The leaves all parties free to work together online.

Different kinds of relatives help in different ways. The parents of young children can be highly motivated to learn technology that helps their children and will often scour online forums about the latest research. The elderly are more technology literate than many give them credit for, with those over 65 years of age spending on average 42 hours per month online in the UK (Ofcom 2007). This is 4 hours more than the next group of users, those whose age is between 18 and 24. The elderly will also learn how to use software, and the experience of the US Department of Veterans Affairs is that patients do work online with clinicians, even though these patients tend to be more elderly, poor, and rural than the rest of the population is (Darkins et al. 2008).

At Patients Know Best, we speak of the family chief medical officer (fCMO). She, and it is more often a "she" than a "he," is responsible for the family's health, caring for the generations of the parents and the children. In many cases, she also has a paid job. Her life is busy, and PHRs can help her help your patients (Figure 4.3).

An example that illustrates this nicely is the elderly patient with Alzheimer's disease. His daughter may not be able to attend the appointment, but the patient is unlikely to be good at telling his daughter what happened at his appointment with you. Putting a copy of the notes into a PHR that the daughter can look at means that she can take care of getting the medications

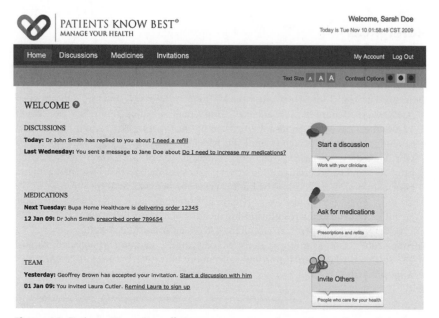

Figure 4.3 Patients Know Best allows everyone to work together online to help the patient, including clinicians and relatives.

that you prescribed and coordinating care with social workers even as she continues her job and looking after her own children.

Unfortunately, the technology literacy of fCMOs tends to be low (Microsoft 2008). They tend to rely on others for computer advice.

But then again, that is why clinical care requires a team. Everyone shares in the goal and the work of improving the patient's health.

Summary box

- New technology requires new techniques.
- PHR technology benefits the whole team, but only if your team adopts new techniques.
- You must train in these new techniques.
- Be selective in the patients with whom you start using PHRs.
- Assume your notes will be read by patients in the future, even if you do not want to start using PHRs today.
- When patients find errors in your notes, thank them, because they are helping you.
- Learn from your patients as they bring new information to your clinical practice.
- Relatives are also helpful, and PHRs solve the traditional technical and legal barriers to making use of their help.

References

Darkins, A., Ryan, P., Kobb, R., Foster, L., Edmonson, E., Wakefield, B., and Lancaster, A.E. , 2008. VA Care Coordination/Home Telehealth Studies 2004–007. *Telemedicine and e-Health* 14(10): 1118–1126.

Doherty, D., 2008. Interview with David Doherty from 3G Doctor. *Patients Know Best podcast.* [Online] Available at: http://podcast.patientsknowbest.com/2008/12/06/interview-with-david-doherty-from-3g-doctor/ [Accessed August 22, 2009].

e-Patient Dave, 2009. Imagine someone had been managing your data, and then you looked. *e-patients.net.* [Online] (Published April 10, 2009) Available at: http://e-patients.net/archives/2009/04/imagine-if-someone-had-been-managing-your-data-and-then-you-looked.html [Accessed August 22, 2009].

Microsoft, 2008. *Copernican Shift.* [Online] (Published June 18, 2008) Available at: http://download.microsoft.com/download/0/4/9/0498CECF-D0B1-4A72-B9B7-17EB7D7ADA98/Copernican_Shift.ppsx [Accessed August 22, 2009].

Ofcom, 2007. The Communications Market 2007. [Online] (Published August 23, 2007) Available at: http://www.ofcom.org.uk/research/cm/cmr07/ [Accessed August 22, 2009].

CHAPTER 5
Educating patients

Without the computer and therefore the printer, broadband and so on, [...] I would just be another dependent person being treated in residential, or day, care doing basket weaving. Social care policy would have most likely be stunted as true individual living would simply not been possible.

Simon Stevens, independent usability trainer and consultant (Stevens 2009)

Patients are motivated to learn by themselves, and it is not your responsibility to teach them. However, as you are reading this book, a little teaching from you can make a big difference to patients. It also establishes for your patients the ways in which you prefer to work online.

Patients are waiting for your encouragement

Patients will not sign up for a new way of working with you unless they believe that you have already signed up as well. If you put a leaflet out in the reception area to test out demand, you will get close to zero uptake. This is not just because few people read the leaflets, but because by relegating the effort to leaflets you are sending out the message that you are doing this half-heartedly.

So if you do this, you have to do it with commitment. After a few months, if things do not work out, you can always go back. For example, if very few patients take up the new services, then it will not be a problem to cancel these services as so few people will be affected. Nor do you have to spend lots of money rolling out all new services simultaneously. You can start slowly by offering to work with your patients using free sites such as PatientsLikeMe.com or RareShare.org.

But whatever you decide you want to start with, you must promote it. Leaflets in the waiting area are useful, but so are letters that go to the homes of patients you think would be suitable, and a leaflet that you give out at the end of each consultation. Posters, kiosks, and websites are all useful in reinforcing the message, but the message itself is you telling the patient in person that you care about the service.

Personal Health Records: A Guide for Clinicians, 1st edition. By Mohammad Al-Ubaydli. Published 2011 by Blackwell Publishing Ltd.

Informing consent: test your patient's comprehension

Not that everyone should use personal health record (PHR) technology. Some patients do not want the responsibility, others do not like computers, and others still do not want to think about their health. You do not need to spend time convincing them of the needs for PHRs. But for patients with long-term illnesses who are committed to improving their health, working with you online is a powerful tool that you should bring to their attention. It is important that you inform these patients before they can consent to working online.

The book's website has useful resources you can download and customize at http://wiki.patientsknowbest.com/Informing_consent. There are two principles: background reading and competency testing.

The first step is to provide the patient with materials explaining the new services you are offering. This is usually available from the different companies whose products you are using, for example, the company that sold you the electronic health record and the patient portal to go with it. Ask each of the companies to provide you with a word document version of their training materials, so you can combine them all into a single document with your institution's logo. Some of them already provide this information in the form of web pages that you can link to, or copy from and paste into your word document. But you should ask them for word documents instead of PDFs, and refuse any paper printouts.

Legally, the next step is to consent the patients. But ethically, it is important to also test their understanding. So, a good way to proceed is to include a comprehension test in the consent form, something we do with all of our patients at Patients Know Best.

The good news is that there is not much you need to seek permission from the patient. Rather than those long Health Insurance Portability and Accountability Act (HIPAA) contracts that explain that you must share data with lots of other parties to do your work for your patients, all you are checking for with a PHR is that the patient agrees for you to enter data about them online in a system that they control.

To confirm that consent is informed, check that the patients understand the implications of the control that they have. Including a questionnaire in the consent form reminds the patient that they are going to see their clinical data before they see their doctor, that they have a responsibility to store their passwords safely, that the internet can never be 100% secure, and that parents do not have unlimited access to their children's records. You can also include reminders of local contacts they have for technical questions or any complaints they have about the service.

Let each patient take the test as many times as they want until they provide all the right answers. The test is as much to give the patient time to reflect on the implications as it is to protect you legally from any misunderstandings that patients have about the service. But once the patients have passed the test and signed the consent forms, you can be sure that you have a cohort of informed and engaged patients, ones who are serious about taking control of their health.

Identifying resources: curation over creation

These patients will use Google to search for information about their illnesses. You will not like everything they find. A common complaint from clinicians is patients who come in clutching stacks of printouts. Clinicians do not have time to read the printouts, nor do they trust many of the websites that patients bring.

The problem is not the website that patients choose, it is that they had to choose alone because you did not choose with them. Even when they look at scientific, peer-reviewed papers in medical journals, patients may well have come across an isolated paper in a weak journal that is not supported by the rest of the literature. Again, the problem is not that the patient is looking at papers without a scientific education, it is that you have not explained to the patient which journals and authors you trust.

Of course, you do not have time to write down everything you know, anymore than you have time to read the printouts from your patients.

Instead, you should curate. On your website, list websites that you trust, ones like the Mayo Clinic (www.mayoclinic.com), WebMD (www.webmd.com), NHS Choices (www.nhs.uk), and MedlinePlus (www.medlineplus.gov). Explain to your patients that you are happy discussing with them any information that they find from these sites because you trust these sites, whereas you cannot spend time checking the accuracy of other sites. Further, explain that the content of the sites you trust of is based on proven medical orthodoxy rather than newer techniques that have not yet had enough testing to prove them.

You can go a step further with tools such as Google custom search engine (www.google.com/cse). Google allows you to create a limited search engine that only searches the websites that you have chosen. The list of sites can be as long as you want, so you can include smaller sites that are relevant to your speciality, or those with local care information. You can then make your custom search engine site available to your patients and say that you will trust any results that the patient gets from searching there.

This example in Figure 5.1 is of creating a custom search for patients with primary immune deficiencies.

Signing up is straightforward, but there are two tricky parts to pay attention to. First, make sure that you select the option "only sites I select" so that the patient only gets results from the sites you preselect.

Next, make sure that you enter the websites that you trust, but leave out the "www." at the beginning. For example, instead of "www.niaid.nih.gov" for the National Institute of Allergy and Infectious Diseases's (NIAID) website, use "niaid.nih.gov." This is because for many websites the "www" prefix changes for different parts of the site. In the case of NIAID, some of the pages

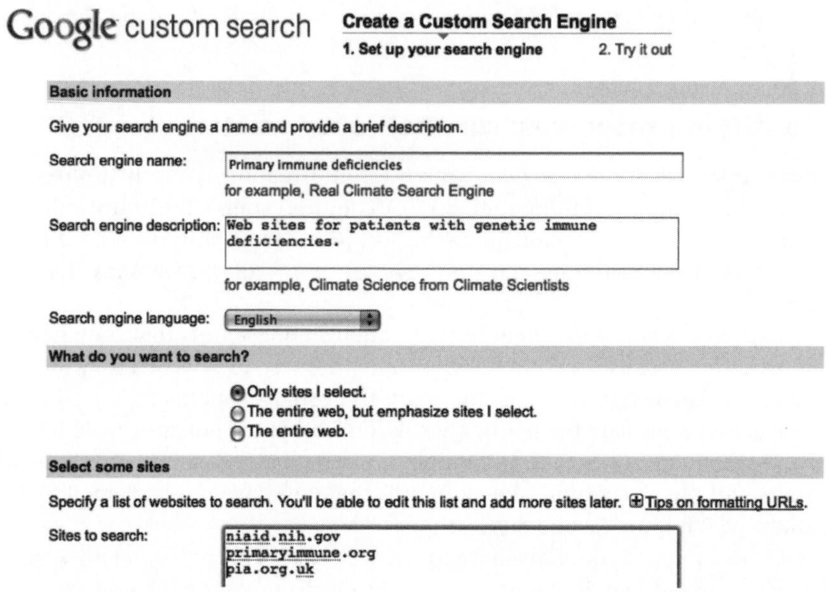

Figure 5.1 Using Google custom search engine to create a custom search for patients with primary immune deficiencies.

are at www3.niaid.nih.gov. If you found this distinction tediously boring, you are correct, and that is why you should leave out the "www." prefix. It means you do not have to worry about these details.

Once you have completed the form, you get two useful things: a link and a widget. The link to your search engine is easy to add to your website, and when the patient clicks on it, they search using the familiar Google user interface. The widget is a little more fancy as it allows you to include the Google user interface inside your own website. This is easy to do—it would take 5 minutes of work from the person who manages your website—but also means that Google advertising appears on your website.

Either way you now have a website that is helpful to your patients as well as keeping them away from unhelpful websites. To see the difference, look at the results of searching on "hyper IgM syndrome" using the above primary immune deficiencies search engine (Figure 5.2).

Compare this with searching in normal Google (Figure 5.3). The Primary Immunodeficiency Association's results are higher in the custom search engine, and those of the National Institutes of Health much higher, than they are with Google's standard search engine.

Turning your patients into data gatherers

Now you can start asking your patients to help you with your information needs. First is the documentation of what happens when they are with other

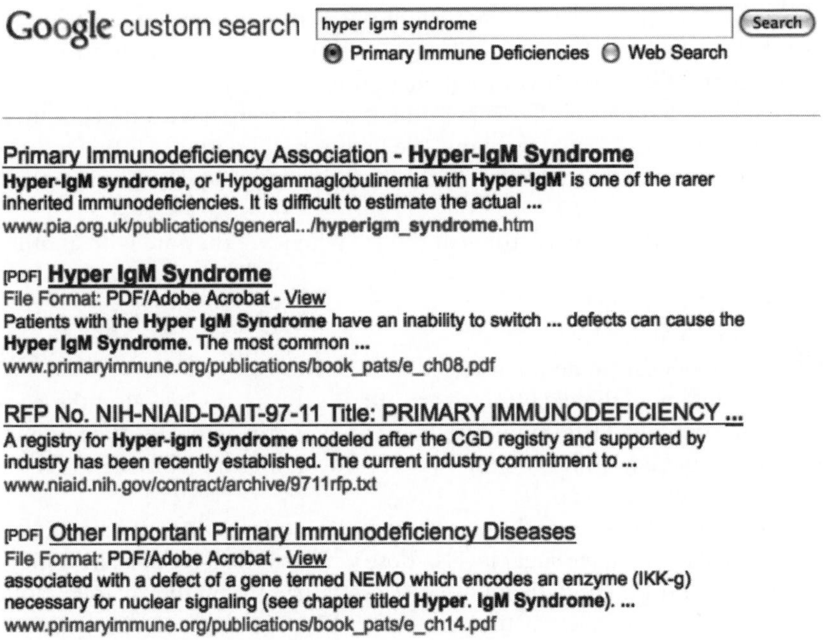

Google custom search | hyper igm syndrome | (Search)

⦿ Primary Immune Deficiencies ◯ Web Search

Primary Immunodeficiency Association - Hyper-IgM Syndrome
Hyper-IgM syndrome, or 'Hypogammaglobulinemia with **Hyper-IgM**' is one of the rarer inherited immunodeficiencies. It is difficult to estimate the actual ...
www.pia.org.uk/publications/general.../**hyperigm_syndrome**.htm

[PDF] Hyper IgM Syndrome
File Format: PDF/Adobe Acrobat - View
Patients with the **Hyper IgM Syndrome** have an inability to switch ... defects can cause the **Hyper IgM Syndrome**. The most common ...
www.primaryimmune.org/publications/book_pats/e_ch08.pdf

RFP No. NIH-NIAID-DAIT-97-11 Title: PRIMARY IMMUNODEFICIENCY ...
A registry for **Hyper-igm Syndrome** modeled after the CGD registry and supported by industry has been recently established. The current industry commitment to ...
www.niaid.nih.gov/contract/archive/9711rfp.txt

[PDF] Other Important Primary Immunodeficiency Diseases
File Format: PDF/Adobe Acrobat - View
associated with a defect of a gene termed NEMO which encodes an enzyme (IKK-g) necessary for nuclear signaling (see chapter titled **Hyper. IgM Syndrome**). ...
www.primaryimmune.org/publications/book_pats/e_ch14.pdf

Figure 5.2 Searching on "hyper IgM syndrome" using a primary immune deficiencies Google custom search engine.

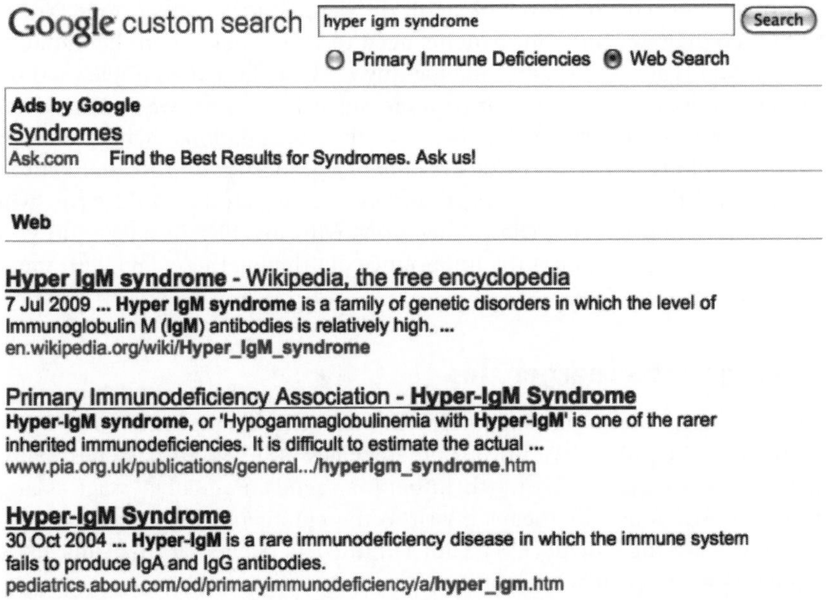

Google custom search | hyper igm syndrome | (Search)

◯ Primary Immune Deficiencies ⦿ Web Search

Ads by Google
Syndromes
Ask.com   Find the Best Results for Syndromes. Ask us!

Web

Hyper IgM syndrome - Wikipedia, the free encyclopedia
7 Jul 2009 ... **Hyper IgM syndrome** is a family of genetic disorders in which the level of Immunoglobulin M (**IgM**) antibodies is relatively high. ...
en.wikipedia.org/wiki/**Hyper_IgM_syndrome**

Primary Immunodeficiency Association - Hyper-IgM Syndrome
Hyper-IgM syndrome, or 'Hypogammaglobulinemia with **Hyper-IgM**' is one of the rarer inherited immunodeficiencies. It is difficult to estimate the actual ...
www.pia.org.uk/publications/general.../**hyperigm_syndrome**.htm

Hyper-IgM Syndrome
30 Oct 2004 ... **Hyper-IgM** is a rare immunodeficiency disease in which the immune system fails to produce IgA and IgG antibodies.
pediatrics.about.com/od/primaryimmunodeficiency/a/**hyper_igm**.htm

Figure 5.3 Searching on "hyper IgM syndrome" using the normal Google search engine.

clinicians. The short-term importance of this is that usually your patient arrives before the letter from the colleague does, if it arrives at all. It is frustrating for both of you when your patient cannot tell you what happened and you have to schedule another appointment for after you have found out from your colleague what really went on. The long-term importance is that by asking your patient to pay attention to the consultation, they also pay attention to their health.

Teach your patients to ask three questions whenever they are with another clinician:

1 What are we doing?
2 Why are we doing it?
3 What happens if we do not do it?

Ask that they note the details in their PHR as soon as possible after the consultation. Using the PHR is important because you can access the data online, or have the patient print it off for your records, rather than having to retype what the patient tells you.

Patients with long-term illnesses should also be gathering other data. Patients with diabetes have sugar levels, those with asthma have peak flow measurements, and others with multiple sclerosis have symptom diaries. Your patients can manually enter the data into PHRs. Consumer devices increasingly come with software that automates the data entry. If you explain to your patients the importance of gathering data, they will surprise you with the devices they find.

You will not have time to look at all the data your patients gather. Nor is it your job to do so. But your patients need to know that, when the moment is right, you really will spend time looking at the data. For example, you do not need to look at each of your patients' sugar levels each week. But when one of these patients comes for their diabetes consultation, spend a minute together looking at their previous results. If you do not do this, the patient will stop wasting their time collecting data. But if you do do this, you will stop wasting time making clinical decisions with insufficient data. And you will have taught the patient the importance of bringing these data with them to all their appointments.

Dealing with emergencies

Perhaps the most important appointment is the emergency one.

Online consultations are not for emergencies: if a patient has chest pain, they need to see a clinician quickly rather than send an e-mail message asking what to do. This usually means a visit to the emergency department. However, the faster the patient sees a clinician, the less likely that that clinician is familiar with the patient's history.

This is when a PHR becomes vital. The patient should bring a printout with their details, as well as the username and password for the website that has their PHR. The printout is important because most clinicians will want to file a printout into the temporary paper notes rather than first learning how to use a new website into their existing workflow. The username and password are important when these clinicians come back to the patient and ask for more clinical details. The patient will either be unconscious, or they will not know the login details as they have to rely on their personal computer to have saved these details. Having them on a piece of paper is a relief during the stress of the emergency department.

And of course, when they finish their visit, hopefully cured and cared for, make sure they write down what happened into the PHR. You will need to look at this when they come to your office the following week.

> **Summary box**
>
> - Education is an important part of the care you provide to patients, and patients are keen to learn.
> - Patients need your encouragement to invest their time in using PHRs to improve their understanding of their health.
> - Test your patients' understanding of PHR technology before you agree to use PHRs with them.
> - Patients need you to identify useful educational resources, but you do not need to create these resources.
> - With a little teaching, patients can bring you all sorts of useful data.
> - PHRs help clinicians who are not familiar with your patients' conditions, for example, during emergencies.

Reference

Stevens, S., 2009. My PC means everything to me as a disabled person. [Online] (Updated January 28, 2009) Available at: http://www.communitycare.co.uk/blogs/social-care-experts-blog/2009/01/by-simon-stevensthe-benefits-t.html   [Accessed July 27, 2010].

CHAPTER 6
Saving time in your clinic

> The first rule of any technology used in a business is that automation applied to an efficient operation will magnify the efficiency. The second is that automation applied to an inefficient operation will magnify the inefficiency.
>
> Bill Gates, founder of Microsoft, and the Bill & Melinda Gates Foundation

There is no way that you will save time with personal health records (PHRs) unless you stop doing some old things you currently do. Because PHRs will require you to spend time doing new things you currently do not do. Setting up your computer, tracking the consent forms your patients signed, giving the patients their passwords, using websites with your patients—all these tasks are new and take time. Furthermore, although the chapter on financial matters discusses some ways in which you can offset the upfront investments you have to make to offer these new services to your patients, there are still new operational costs. Unless you get rid of some old costs, you will just keep them and add new ones.

Most clinicians say that they understand this. They nod and say that they want technology to make their work more efficient. However, they act differently. They do not eliminate follow-up appointments because they worry about liability. They insist on looking at all test results, even the majority that are normal, rather than just the ones that need attention. They do not send advice electronically because they think patients cannot use computers. And they do not have telephone consultations because they do not know how to start doing so.

This chapter is to help you start. It is hard because it requires you to get rid of old habits. It is scary because your colleagues will continue with their old habits. But it is worth it.

Study yourself

Dr. Richard Smith, former editor of the *British Medical Journal*, accompanied his mother to her appointment with an orthopedic surgeon. This was a post-operative follow-up appointment, and his mother had recovered well. It was

Personal Health Records: A Guide for Clinicians, 1st edition. By Mohammad Al-Ubaydli.
Published 2011 by Blackwell Publishing Ltd.

a 1-hour trip to the specialist and a 2-hour wait in the clinic as it inevitably overran. Once inside, it took the surgeon a couple of minutes to confirm that Richard's mother was indeed doing well, starting with the fact that she had walked into the room.

Why, asked Richard, did the surgeon need a face-to-face appointment to confirm this? Why not limit the consultation to a telephone where a health professional asks his mother how she is doing? Better still, why not give the patient a list of reasons to call the surgeon's team, or the family physician, and eliminate follow-up for all other patients?

At your next clinic session, try this exercise. After each appointment, write down the problem that the patient came with and what would stop you from doing the appointment over the telephone instead of in person.

There are lots of reasons to avoid using the phone for appointments. Some of these are even good ones. For example, an examination of a patient's abdomen is important in acute abdominal pain. But the point of this exercise is to find cases when there is no good reason.

Switch to telephone calls

Patients who call Dr. Tony Stern's office asking for an appointment are offered a call- back from him within 2 hours. When he calls them, usually on their cell phone, he takes a full history. For about one-third of these calls, the patient just wants advice, for example, about an over-the-counter medication that the patient can get, or a sick note that Dr. Stern writes straight away. For another third, the call is a consultation, discussing the implications of test results that he has received, asking for a referral he begins there, and then, or a prescription that he writes. Many pharmacies already offer home delivery, so these patients do not even need to leave the house.

Finally, another third of patients really do need a face-to-face appointment, and these are offered an appointment within 24 hours. Tony is the only partner in a practice that cares for 4,100 patients. Before his partner's retirement, the two of them cared for 4,000 patients, full-time. You can see a short lecture and video by Tony at http://wiki.patientsknowbest.com/Tony_Stern.

Talk to your team

You cannot make the switch by yourself: your team must commit with you. For example, although you can start with a few call-backs by yourself, if you make the call-backs the default alternative and your receptionist has not understood why, the patient will hear the uncertainty in his or her explanation. The patient will not conclude that they are getting the convenient service of telephone calls, but the lesser service of no face-to-face appointments. If your fellow clinicians are not sure that the switch is safe, they will start scheduling compensatory follow-up appointments for your patients. So although you can start experimenting by yourself, you must discuss with your team what you are finding and why it is good for them to try the same.

It is important in the discussion to explicitly express everyone's fears. Safety is paramount of course: what if you miss something that you would have found on examination? Efficiency is another as the risk is that you start with a telephone call and then find you must call in the patient anyway for the same length of appointment. Then there is the matter of communicating this to patients.

Once you have understood these concerns, you can start overcoming them together. If you are worried about safety, you can do an audit with 100 patients, 50 of whom you help on the phone, and 50 of whom you ask to come for an appointment just as you would have previously. See how many problems you would have failed to pick up if the patients had not come in person. More importantly, see which problems you could pick up over the telephone if you explicitly sought them out. For telephone consultations that have to be converted into face-to-face appointments, see if you can find new processes that would eliminate this. Finally, you must be careful how you communicate new workflow to patients.

Talk to your patients

Patients must not think you are making it harder to have face-to-face appointments, and instead insisting on telephone and online consultations. Partly this is because they will not like what looks like a reduction in service. But most importantly, if patients do not feel they can book an appointment, you cannot feel safe in telling them to call you for a follow-up.

Make the appointments available, and make sure each patient gets the appointment with the clinician who originally spoke to them about the problem.

But once you have these safeguards in place, you can comfortably advertise the benefits of the new service. The key is to understand that, for the patient, a 10-minute appointment means half a day off work. He or she must travel to your office, find a parking spot, often wait beyond the appointment as clinics run late, and then travel back. The minutes add up to a lot of inefficiency for the patient.

In the United States and other countries with private health care systems, the lower costs of telephone and online consultations can be passed onto patients as lower fees and co-pays. The chapter on finance goes through examples of US health insurance companies who have understood and shared the benefits with their patients, but you can get started with small trials with your patients paying directly.

For example, private physician customers of Patients Know Best can charge patients directly for online consultations at prices that suit their population. This allows the physicians to better serve patients who have jobs, or the patient's relatives who cannot attend the appointment with the patient but still need to work with the clinical team to look after the patient.

Online consultations

As with telephone consultations, online ones are best done simply at first. For example, Cisco's care-at-a-distance solutions are extraordinary for their power and sophistication (http://www.cisco.com/web/strategy/healthcare/care_at_a_distance.html). However, they also require a large financial investment upfront, and both you and the patient need to use specialized Cisco devices. Furthermore, the devices try to replicate the existing face-to-face consultations with both you and the patient talking through the video cameras at the same time. Many other telemedicine initiatives have also taken the same expensive approach, although Cisco is perhaps one of the best efforts so far.

At Patients Know Best, we took the opposite approach, focusing on simplicity. Many clinicians already receive e-mails from their patients, or at least requests from patients to be allowed to send e-mails. Far more patients and clinicians already have access to e-mail than will ever have access to high-definition video cameras. Furthermore, the asynchronous nature of e-mail is a strength, not a weakness. In other words, patients who already know you, and understand their illness, would like to send occasional messages asking specific questions. They would often like to do so from their office, where they do not want anyone else to hear them discuss their clinical details, or outside of your office hours, when they would like to send the question and resume whatever they were doing. They are happy waiting for you to respond within 24 hours, just as they are used to your office's response after leaving a voicemail message.

Of course, you cannot use normal e-mail for clinical consultations because the technology that most patients use is not secure, and does not comply with the auditing regulations that most countries have for clinical documentation. So our software provides a website that both you and the patient can use to send messages to each other securely. As both you and the patients gain trust in the system, you can invest more time and effort in adding features. For example, our software can integrate with your local e-mail system to guarantee secure delivery of messages so that you do not even need to log into the website. Integrating with your laboratory system allows sending test results directly to patients through the website or their cell phones. Ultimately, the entire medical record can be shared through our PHR.

But each of these should only be attempted after the earlier attempt had proved useful and popular. And each attempt should be adapted to fit your existing workflow. For example, the first immunology team to use our software had the same specialist nurse who had checked voicemail daily also check the website to answer patients' online consultation questions. Other customers had their care coordinator carry out this task, while another physician liked to log into the website herself every day.

Sending information online

You and your team spend a lot of time on sending information to patients. Whether it is printing off letters, licking envelopes, calling patients, or giving them printouts during an appointment, a lot of work is involved. The UK's National Health Service requires specialists to send a summary letter to both the patient and the primary care physician at the end of each consultation.

The scale of work is an order of magnitude greater when it comes to screening programs. For example, England's colon cancer screening is handled by several regional centers, each of which mails fecal occult blood testing kits to people over the age of 60, and then mails the test results to those who submit their stool samples. And because regional specialists are doing the work, bypassing local primary care physicians, worried patients with further questions about the meaning of their test results like to ask the specialists directly.

Online delivery of information saves a lot of time, money, and anxiety. You can minimize time because printing off letters and sending them to the right patient are a manual and error-prone process. Physical delivery is more expensive than electronic delivery. And anxiety can be reduced with PHR software because the electronic delivery can include interactive links to further information, and direct online consultations with the person who best understands each patient's results.

The logistics of switching to online communication are complicated and expensive, however, so you should only attempt this after achieving early successes with the other tools discussed in this chapter. The complexity is from technology integration, ensuring security of communication, and allowing patient choice. And the expense is from the integration. But PHRs are the secret.

In the United States, PHRs include Google Health, Microsoft HealthVault, and Patients Know Best. The appendix has instruction manuals that you can give to your patients so they learn how to use the former, while our website has videos for our own software. But the tools that Google and Microsoft provide to clinicians are limited. Instead, you must connect your electronic health record (EHR) to these PHRs. It is important to connect to both as your patients will want to choose the one they prefer. But your IT staff will struggle with each connection. That is why the Patients Know Best platform was designed to allow your EHR to connect to both of their PHRs, and to those of others, so that the patient can choose where to receive their data.

The hardest part about security is making sure that the person who claims to be communicating with you using the PHR is actually the patient you are supposed to be working with. This is why you must insist on seeing photographic identification when a patient first registers to use the software with you, and why Patients Know Best integrates tracking of identification into administrative tools.

Once you have cleared these hurdles, you can tell your patients that you are ready to send them information online. Not everyone will be ready, at first. But in banking, electronic delivery of statements has steadily risen over the past few years, and 55% of those who bank online have also opted to stop paper delivery (Higdon and Davis 2009). And patients like using their mobile phones to receive test results (Menon-Johansson et al. 2006) because of speed, and because their phones feel private and intimate. Finally, the administrative tools of Patients Know Best software allow patients to nominate family members to access their results online even when the patients cannot or do not want to use the internet.

All these trends mean that you can create new processes which automate efficiency and raise the quality of care for your patients. The following chapters will cover the technical, legal, and financial details of making these possibilities into realities.

Summary box

- You will only benefit from the new technology of PHRs if you get rid of some of your old habits.
- Study the appointments you have to see which did not need to happen face-to-face.
- Switch some of these appointments to telephone calls, and others to PHRs.
- Your whole clinical team has to agree with this approach for it to succeed in saving time and raising quality.
- Your patients also have to agree, so they see this change as service improvement rather than cost-cutting.
- Online delivery of information saves a lot of time, money, and anxiety.
- Online consultations can save time and increase revenues.

References

Higdon, E. and Davis, E., 2009. The time has come to eliminate paper statements. *Forrester* July 17.

Menon-Johansson, A.S., McNaught, F., Mandalia, S., and Sullivan, A.K., 2006. Texting decreases the time to treatment for genital *Chlamydia trachomatis* infection. *Sexually Transmitted Infections* 82(1): 49–51.

PART 3
Your practice

CHAPTER 7

Technology

> May all your problems be technical.
>
> Dr. Jim Gray, winner of the Turing Award, the "Nobel prize of
> computer science"

I am always surprised when a clinician describes himself or herself as a technophobe. Medicine is full of technology, and clinicians love using this technology to help patients. Anesthetics and antibiotics, endoscopes and stethoscopes, vaccines, and x-rays—technology is everywhere. And then there are the process technologies: from the healing of nursing to the peace of hospices, the humble Heimlich Maneuver, and the daily death-defying acts of resuscitation.

Information technology (IT) is the next wave of innovation, arriving just in time to help professionals whose daily work is built around information. It is not that hard to understand, at least, not for someone who has already mastered the difficult concepts of health care. But it will be increasingly hard to provide patient care without understanding IT. So this chapter is in two parts. The first is a short introduction to the basic concepts of IT, so you can share it with colleagues who are new to personal health records (PHRs). And the second part explains PHR technology and how you can deploy it in your institution for your patients. If there is one thing I can urge you to do, it is to outsource your IT work. It is important to have someone in-house who coordinates all the IT work. But the more that person outsources IT work, the better for you, and this chapter aims to give you some of the education to do so.

IT 101

There are only four building blocks in IT: data, hardware, software, and networks. Every term you hear from IT professionals is either an example of these terms or a combination of them:

1 Data are information, for example, a patient's sugar results from this morning, their x-ray image from last week, or your message discussing the two.
2 Hardware is a physical device, for example, a computer, laptop, or telephone.

Personal Health Records: A Guide for Clinicians, 1st edition. By Mohammad Al-Ubaydli. Published 2011 by Blackwell Publishing Ltd.

3 Software is instructions written by a human being to control hardware, for example, PHR software that copies the sugar result from your computer to the patient's phone.

4 A network is a collection of data, hardware, and software, for example, Windows on a computer, Cerner electronic health records on a phone or Patients Know Best's PHRs software.

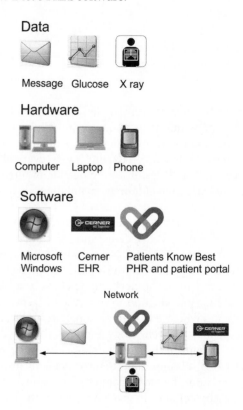

Data

Message   Glucose   X ray

Hardware

Computer   Laptop   Phone

Software

Microsoft   Cerner   Patients Know Best
Windows   EHR   PHR and patient portal

Network

PHR data

Data are only useful if software is able to work with the data. This in turn is determined by the format of the data, that is, the way in which the data are organized. For example, if you think of a medical history on a piece of paper, it is usually organized by headings: presenting complaint, history of presenting complaint, and past medical history. If you changed the sequence of headings, or even wrote in free text without any headings at all, your colleagues would still be able to make sense of what you wrote. A computer would not. Computers are very literal, and software only works if data points appear in the same sequence under the same headings. The format of the data is crucial.

The most important PHR data formats are continuity of care record (CCR) and continuity of care document (CCD). They organize data in a similar way to a referral letter, listing all pertinent information about the patient, including current problems, past medical history, medications, and allergies.

In the United States, most PHR software supports the CCR, and many support the CCD as well. For example, the PHR software of Google, Microsoft, and Patients Know Best can send and receive data in the CCR format. Microsoft also supports CCD. Pharmacies such as Walgreens and CVS and providers such as MinuteClinic also support CCR. If you are interested, you can read more of the technical details at wiki.patientsknowbest.com/CCR, but you do not need to.

What you *do* need to do, however, is to choose software that supports CCR and CCD. This support allows you to send data from your software to the PHR software that your patients want to use. Because these standards are new, none of your old software will support them. However, new software can include support, so you should always check for this, and demand proof that there will be support in the future if the software vendor says the current software does not do so already. And you should start asking the creators of your old software for upgrades to support CCR and CCD. It takes a while to include support in an upgrade, so the sooner you start asking, the better.

PHR hardware

There are three kinds of hardware: yours, the patient's, and the hardware that connects yours to the patient's.

You do not need any special or new hardware for PHRs. Carry on with the same computers you already own, but also consider that most modern phones are powerful computers. So your BlackBerry, iPhone, or other smartphones can be useful for working with PHRs while on the move, especially for receiving and responding to patients' messages.

Neither does your patient need any special or new hardware. Most PHRs simply require a web browser, for example, Internet Explorer or Firefox, which means that any computer from the last 3 years is already powerful enough. However, although modern phones can access these websites, their screens are usually too small to show all the data clearly. It is better to recommend that the patient uses a computer with a large screen. Note that the patient does not need to own the computer as they can use one in their local library instead.

The connecting hardware is what your IT team should worry about. For a patient portal, they will set up and maintain a powerful computer that shares all your data with your patients through a website. For a web PHR, your IT team will rely on the immensely powerful hardware of the PHR providers such as Google, Microsoft, or Patients Know Best.

One thing you should avoid, and your IT department will try to prevent, is connecting your hardware directly to your patients'. This is because the connection makes it easy to spread computer viruses. Direct connections are necessary for PHRs that store a patient's data locally on their computer or USB drive. The designers of these local PHRs take this approach because data are more difficult to attack if they are stored locally than if they are stored on the internet. On the other hand, it is easier for a computer virus to attack your own computer if you directly connect the patient's computer.

If you really do want to support direct connections, the safest way to do this is through having a separate computer in your institution to which the patient can connect theirs. That is safer than sharing information directly on the internet, and you can also wall off that computer from spreading viruses accidentally transmitted from patients' computers.

PHR software

In 10 years, most clinicians will be using PHR software with their patients. Each patient and clinician will get there through a different route.

In the short term, the early adopters will be patients who invite their clinicians to work online. These are patient-led PHR deployments, and for most of these, all that the clinician needs is a web browser to use the PHR website that the patient chose. A few patient-led PHR tools require the clinician to install special software, but for the most part you should avoid these because they require too much of your time for too few of your patients.

But web-based patient-led PHR software is worth embracing. Not only is this a good way to help patients who are truly committed to improving their health, it is also the easiest way to understand PHR technology. Your patient will gladly teach you how to use the software, and for the most part, web-based PHRs are designed to quickly deliver time savings. Once you have learned how to use the software, you can approach your institution about a clinician-led PHR, because in the long term, clinician-led PHRs are the most likely route to mainstream adoption. Not only do you hold a lot of data that make a PHR useful, most patients will not use a PHR unless they know that you will use it with them.

You will need to work with three types of software. First, you need to use electronic health records (EHRs) in your daily practice. If you are not entering clinical data on a computer, there is nothing to share with your patients' PHRs. So make sure you have a good EHR system and that your clinical team is using it. *Finding the right EHR*, the sister book to this one, provides an excellent guide to get you started (Gasch and Gasch 2010).

Second, you need a patient portal to make your EHR data available outside of your institution, that is, to patients. Increasingly, EHR vendors provide a patient portal add-on. If you are considering EHR vendors, make sure that either they already support a patient portal or they have plan to do so in the near future. Patient portals may not be common now, but your competitor will likely have one while you still have the same EHR as you currently do.

It is easier to choose an EHR provider with a patient portal than to switch to one that does, so start by demanding the correct tools from your vendors.

Third, you need to connect to the PHR of your patients. This is hard and requires computer professionals. As a clinician what you must do is insist that the data transfer is through the CCR as this is the data standard that your patient portal must support.

In the United States, the two commonest PHR platforms to support are Microsoft HealthVault and Google Health. The appendix has more information about each of these. In the long run it is important to support both. In the beginning, however, your institution will likely begin by supporting one. For example, the Mayo Clinic integrates with Microsoft HealthVault, while the Cleveland Clinic integrates with Google Health. Because both Microsoft and Google are offering support data exchange through the CCR, your team can relatively easily support the second platform after doing the hard work of supporting the first.

It is possible to go directly from EHR to PHR. This is what my company, Patients Know Best, offers in its software. Our patient portal connects to most EHR software, as well as acting as a PHR in its own right.

Collecting data from patients

Patients have even more data to give to you than you have to give to them. Glucose meters, peak flow devices, oximeters, and 24-hour ECG recorders are all examples of devices that increasingly have computer chips inside them. And once a device is digital, it can share data with other digital devices, for example, your computer.

The secret is the Continua data standard (www.continuaalliance.org). Originally created by Intel®, it has been embraced by a large number of organizations including Bayer, GE, Kaiser Permanente, and Partners Healthcare. Nor is it a purely American standard as the UK's National Health Service and Spain's Clinic Barcelona are also members. What is most interesting for the future is the number of consumer brands that have joined, including Nokia, Panasonic, and Samsung.

Right now, only a few devices feed directly into PHRs. For example, Omron Healthcare (www.omronhealthcare.com) makes a pedometer and a blood pressure monitor that connect directly to Microsoft HealthVault.

But over the next 5 years, many more devices will be available in the market. If your institution bulk-buys devices for patients, make sure the purchasing committee knows about the importance of the standard as a factor in choosing between devices. If your patients buy the devices directly, make sure they know to look for the logo and compatibility. And the next time a sales representative comes to tell you about their company's product line, tell them how important the standard is to your work with patients.

Regional data networks

Governments around the world have led efforts to electronically share clinical data across institutions. Sharing clinical data is important to save time, money, and lives. It is essential for safe clinical practice. Electronic sharing should be faster, cheaper, and more accurate than doing so with paper. So these regional efforts are laudable.

In the United States, Regional Health Information Organizations (RHIOs) are regional groupings to support data sharing. Hospitals in a geographic region would work together with an RHIO to set up a health information exchange (HIE). The HIE would allow data to move between all members in the region, and ultimately, data would move between different RHIOs' HIEs. In England, the National Health Service set up five clusters, equivalent to US HIEs, each of which would share data through a single national network, the NHS Spine.

However, in most countries the early attempts have failed to meet their ambitious aims. Partly, this is because of the sheer size of their ambitions, but is also because of their centralized approach. Health care, for better or worse, is distributed across many institutions, and centralizing their data is hard. Furthermore, it raises so many privacy issues that the compensatory privacy protections raise barriers and costs. Finally, in countries with private health systems such as in the United States, institutions in the same region found it difficult to share data with their competitors.

For all these reasons, PHRs may well be the best way to share data. Giving a copy of their data to each patient is less ambitious than storing all patients' data in one central system. It also avoids many privacy problems, and it means sharing data with customers rather than competitors.

Outsource your IT department

So now you know about all these enormous national efforts, what can your small team do? My advice is that, as much as possible, you should outsource your IT department. You already outsource the development, storage, and distribution of medicines, devices, and transportation. You should do the same to fulfill your information technology needs. This is not just to save money, but also to raise quality. Your IT department should focus on choosing the best technology providers and managing their contracts just as your pharmacists choose the best medicines and manage their suppliers.

There are many advantages to doing this. The most obvious is specialization. For example, your IT team will likely only ever set up one patient portal. If you use an outside company to set up and manage the portal, however, you can be sure that their staff will have far more experience than your own internal staff does. Their expertise at keeping patient data safe is much greater than your own team's.

Specialization also allows economies of scale. Providing centralized computing infrastructure to ten hospitals is cheaper, per hospital, than for each hospital to create their own data center locally. The same economies of scale mean that you rely on electricity from your local power station, rather than your hospital's generator (Carr 2008).

A more subtle reason is financial. As health care institutions invest more in information technology, they have raised capital budgets, to allow the increased purchases. But operating budgets have not kept pace (HIMSS Analytics 2008), meaning that IT departments have struggled to provide enough support for ever more hardware, software, and data. Outsourcing maintenance makes it easier to identify costs, measure benefits, and switch to different providers to get better value.

Most importantly, working with outside providers means getting access to best practices. This is because, as independent specialists, these companies embed the best working habits into their software based on their experience with all the other health care institutions they work with. The best practices you have read about in this book on working with patients online are embedded into every part of our software at Patients Know Best.

The past few years have seen a flowering of outsourcing options. For example, at the start of 2009, Dell, Walmart, and eClinicalWorks collaborated to provide an EHR solution at a low price and with ongoing maintenance (www.dell.com/emr). American Well (www.americanwell.com), Hello Health (www.hellohealth.com), and Patients Know Best—all provide and manage software for online consultations.

The secret to letting go, however, is holding onto the data. Creating data about your patients is one of the most valuable things you do for them. It is vital that you, and not your IT provider, control these data. Control does not require that the data to remain physically in your building. In fact, most hospitals today cannot move data from the EHR software inside their building to any other software without the help of the EHR software's provider. In these cases, the IT provider is in control of the data, even though the data are inside buildings and computers are owned by the hospital.

Rather, you must be able move the data around to a competitor when you want to do so. Not only does this give you the freedom to move to the best IT provider, it also encourages your existing provider to constantly improve, lest they lose your business.

At Patients Know Best, we ensure this by storing all patient data inside an EHR for which the programming code is available for anyone else to use. This transparency means that any data can be moved to and used by the EHR, patient portal, or PHR of any other company. If your IT vendor does not provide this transparency, you can still insist that their software can prepare all patient data in the CCR format. You should also specify in the contract that the provider will help you with the transfer process if you choose to work with another provider.

Because the opportunities from working with different providers are wonderful ones. Traditionally, health care has invested less in information technology than other industries have (Gartner 2009). But this is not for lack of interest in technology, but rather because it took a while for the information technology industry to create solutions to the unique and complex problems of health care. As these solutions are available to you on the market, you can choose the best ones to provide the best care. Your patients will thank you for it.

Summary box

- Information technology is just one of many technologies that clinicians already adopt to improve patient care.
- The four building blocks are data, hardware, software, and networks.
- PHR data formats include the continuity of care record, whose users include Google, Microsoft, Patients Know Best, CVS, and Walgreens.
- PHR hardware is, for the most part, the hardware you and your patient already have.
- But to connect your hardware to your patients' you should use powerful platforms like those of Google, Microsoft, or Patients Know Best.
- PHR software is easiest and most powerful to use when it is web-based.
- Medical devices are increasingly compatible with PHRs using the Continua standard.
- Regional data networks are promising but disappointing.
- You IT team should focus on buying from the best outsourcers rather than trying to create IT your own information technology.

References

Carr, N., 2008. The big switch. W.W. Norton & Co. Available at: www.nicholasgcarr.com/bigswitch [Accessed July 27, 2010].

Gartner, 2009. *Forecast: Industry Market Strategies by Vertical Industry, Worldwide, 2006–2012, 1Q09 Update*. Stamford: Gartner.

Gasch, A. and Gasch, B., 2010. *Finding the Right EHR: Your Guide to Electronic Health Records Success*. Oxford: Wiley-Blackwell.

HIMSS Analytics, 2008. *2008 Annual Report for the US Hospital Market*. Chicago: Healthcare Information and Management Systems Society.

CHAPTER 8

Law

If a physician make a large incision with the operating knife, and kill [the patient], or open a tumor with the operating knife, and cut out the eye, his hands shall be cut off.

Law 218, the Code of Hammurabi (Codex Hammurabi), 1790 BC,
ancient Babylon (King 1910)

Laws are the binds that set men free. They help humans to trust each other. Take a moment to consider how amazing surgery is. The recovery of the patient after an operation shows how advanced medical care is. The survival of the patient during the operation is a tribute to the skills of the surgical team.

But I am still awed by the patient's willing submission to the surgeon: the trust they place by walking into a room, agreeing to be put to sleep, knowing full well that the surgeon is waiting to cut them with a knife. Mankind is the only species capable of building such trust between a doctor and a patient.

The law is important to building this trust. Only those who have studied in medical school and passed medical examinations are allowed to work as doctors. If a doctor is negligent, they must compensate the patient. And if unethical, they will lose their license to practice. These checks and balances help patients trust doctors, and similar laws govern the work of all clinicians with patients.

Patients (will) own their data

In general, you should assume that patients own data about them, and that clinicians are custodians for the data.

Few countries' laws have adopted this view wholesale, but it makes moral sense and more voters are patients than are clinicians. So around the world in democratic legislatures, the trend is toward this approach. Furthermore, this mindset is patient-friendly, so adopting it early reduces the probability that in the future patients will feel that you have misused their data or breached their privacy.

Personal Health Records: A Guide for Clinicians, 1st edition. By Mohammad Al-Ubaydli.
Published 2011 by Blackwell Publishing Ltd.

Europe

The European Union's laws embody this approach. Its Data Protection Act (Information Commissioner's Office 2008) is easy to understand but hard to follow. With few exemptions, it requires that all personally identifiable data are:

- Fairly and lawfully processed
- Processed for limited purposes
- Adequate, relevant, and not excessive
- Accurate and up to date
- Not kept for longer than is necessary
- Processed in line with your rights
- Secure
- Not transferred to other countries without adequate protection

Compliance is easier with personal health records (PHRs) than with patient portals because the data and their sharing are controlled by the patient rather than the health care institution. For example, because the patient is the one who invites clinicians to access and use their PHR, it is easier to prove that the usage was "processed for limited purposes." The patient is in control of these limitations.

By contrast, the clinical team invites the patient to use their institution's patient portal. So the institution is in control and responsible. Documenting the patient's consent for each act of sharing, when controlled by the institution, is a heavy responsibility.

This legal framework means you can do more when you have less control. So give the patient practical control over the data.

USA

The laws in the United States are a little more complicated as federal legislators take a sectoral approach, with different laws for different sectors. For health care, the Health Insurance Portability and Accountability Act (HIPAA) regulates the disclosure of protected health information (PHI), that is, the movement of data about the patient between institutions that work with the patient. Broadly speaking, HIPAA treats clinical data as the intellectual property of the patient, and the clinicians' note-taking as work-for-hire. And so although the clinician may physically own the piece of paper or the filing cabinet, the clinical data on the paper inside the cabinet are the property of the patient.

There are a couple of important but temporary exceptions. For example, the HIPAA Privacy Rule treats test results as a special case. Instead, regulations of the Centers for Medicare and Medicaid Services state that results can only be delivered to "authorized persons." The current definition does not include the patient who is the subject of the test. The definition is likely to change soon as the campaigns of patient advocacy groups gain momentum (HealthDataRights.org 2009).

At the time of writing, the second exception was about to end: by 2010, HIPAA legislation will apply to PHR vendors. This was not the case when Google and Microsoft launched their PHR products in 2008, but the American Recovery and Reinvestment Act of 2009 (www.recovery.gov) updated HIPAA to fix this omission.

As in Europe this legislation means that PHRs are easier to work with than patient portals are. As soon as your institution "discloses" PHI data to the patient through the patient's chosen PHR, you are no longer responsible for problems with the data in the PHR. The PHR vendor is responsible for documenting that their product always obeyed the orders of the patient, and that there were no breaches of the data center. But your institution is not. A patient portal, by contrast, means that your institution takes on that responsibility.

The responsibility includes breach notification (www.ftc.gov/healthbreach) and is regulated by the Federal Trade Commission (FTC). Institutions that have had a security breach must do the following:

Notify everyone whose information was breached

In many cases, notify the media

Notify the FTC

For an excellent discussion of the details of the FTC's rules, it is worth listening to the podcast interview (Lombardi 2009) with Marc Lombardi, health care expert at the law firm, Brown Rudnick, because these rules also include responsibilities for the patient.

Rights mean responsibilities

To misquote Spider-man, with more rights come more responsibilities. And so as patients demand their data, they are also responsible for making sure that the data are stored securely. The patient must choose wisely which PHR companies to work with.

To help with this, the EU's Data Protection Act and the US Federal Trade Commission have rightly and explicitly tackled the issue of appropriate consent. For example, although HIPAA provides the patient with important rights, many consent forms ask the patient to waive these rights.

But for PHRs the FTC has said that "if a privacy policy contains buried disclosures describing extensive dissemination of consumers' data the patient cannot be said to have authorized such dissemination. Instead the FTC talks about individuals' reasonable expectations" (Federal Trade Commission 2009).

Of course, just because the European Union and FTC demand compliance, and promise punishment, does not mean that patients will not be harmed. Some PHR companies will be incompetent, others will be malicious, and it is an early market. Inevitably, some companies will cause damage until the regulators catch up with them.

So the patient still has to approach PHR companies with care. It is useful to share with patients the checklist at http://wiki.patientsknowbest. com/PHR_vendors. The checklist teaches the patient to ask about the company's team, the claims they make about security, and the policies they publish to support these claims. Nothing can be guaranteed to be safe, but a little work identifies companies that are good to work with, and then you can do good work with your patients.

Summary box

- Medicine is built on trust between the patient and the clinician.
- Medical laws and regulations support building of this trust, as does the increasing ownership by patients of their data.
- The European Union's Data Protection Acts and the US Health Insurance Portability and Accountability Act both state that data about the patient are owned by the patient.
- By handing over control of the data to the patient, you make it easier and more ethical to share data with other clinicians to support safe care.
- Patient rights go hand in hand with patient responsibilities: when a patient chooses they also become responsible for the outcome of the choice.

References

Federal Trade Commission, 2009. 16 CFR Part 318 Health Breach Notification Rule: final rule. [Online] (Created August 25, 2009) Available at: http://edocket.access. gpo.gov/2009/pdf/E9-20142.pdf [Accessed October 27, 2009].

HealthDataRights.org, 2009. Consensus letter to the Office of Civil Rights and the Centers for Medicare and Medicaid Services on the need for expanding the rights of individuals to access their test results. [Online] (Created October 20, 2009) Available at: http://www.healthdatarights.org/pdfs/CLIA-Letter.pdf [Accessed October 21, 2009].

Information Commissioner's Office, 2008. Data Protection Act (DPA)—the basics. [Online] (Created June 17, 2008) Available at: http://www.ico.gov.uk/what_we_cover/ data_protection/the_basics.aspx [Accessed October 27, 2009].

King, L., 1910. Translation of Codex Hammurabi. [Online] (Updated June 6,1999) Available at: http://www.wsu.edu/~dee/MESO/CODE.HTM [Accessed October 26, 2009].

Lombardi, M., 2009. Podcast interview with Marc Lombardi about PHR legislation. [Online] (Created October 14, 2009) Available at: http://podcast. patientsknowbest. com [Accessed October 30, 2009].

CHAPTER 9

Finance

The nine most terrifying words in the English language are: "I'm from the government and I'm here to help".

Ronald Reagan

For the majority of US clinicians without even an electronic health record (EHR), the government is here to help. There are research grants, tax breaks, stimulus funds, and data collection bonuses. But there are also other sources of funds including your own institution's central funds, private payers, and patients. Whatever the source, you must think about payments.

Ask to be paid

There is no point in being shy about this: you must get paid for working online with patients. First, this is the right thing to do. If you are helping patients, you need to be paid for it, just as you are for all the help that you give to patients. Second, unless you are paid, you risk a pay cut as you stop doing work that you are paid for. Third, generating money from this new way of working means you can invest in new resources that support it.

And finally, the payer can hold you accountable. This is crucial for improving the quality of service for patients, and for increasing adoption. Because if no one can prove any benefits to patient experience, any reductions in costs, and any improvements to quality, then it is important that you stop. There are lots of other ways that health care can deliver improvements. Spend time on those instead. But if you count the value for the payer, they will value paying you.

Ask to be paid from the early on. Most likely, your request will be rejected at first. But if you do not ask for it, you will never be paid.

Salaried clinicians

In the United States, the large-scale pioneers of this work have been integrated health care systems such as Community Health Network (www. ecommunity.com), the Department of Veterans Affairs (www.myhealth. va.gov), and Kaiser Permanente. This is because, especially with salaried

Personal Health Records: A Guide for Clinicians, 1st edition. By Mohammad Al-Ubaydli.
Published 2011 by Blackwell Publishing Ltd.

physicians, they could capture the productivity benefits of technology, serving more patients with the same number of clinicians.

Some health systems began their deployments with limited financial incentives in pilots to encourage the clinicians to try out the new technology. This was to counter salaried clinicians' worries that an increased workload would lead to more hours without an increase in pay. However, early data from the pilots have shown such worries to be ill-founded.

Kaiser Permanente in particular has been active in measuring the success of its initiatives, publishing the results of its trials. For example, the March issue of *Health Affairs* is well worth reading and includes a Kaiser paper that shows the shift in patient contacts to telephone and internet consultations (Chen et al. 2009).

In the UK, the market trend is for primary care trusts to expect National Health Service providers to include telephone and internet consultations as part of the overall service that they offer to patients. Customers of Patients Know Best (www.patientsknowbest.com) have already begun using the software to support patients with serious conditions and minimize their travel.

Bupa, the country's largest health insurer, and Great Ormond Street Hospital, its largest children's hospital, use the Patients Know Best personal health record (PHR) to reduce the costs of data sharing across institutions. It is cheaper to give the data to the patient, and have the patient share the data with their different providers of care, than for these providers to transfer the data. The savings rise with the complexity of disease.

There are other financial benefits for health systems. For example, some have been counting the overhead costs of face-to-face consultations. These include the wear and tear on car parks; the salaries of car park attendants, and staff who direct patients to appointments; and the utility costs of lighting, heating, and water. Patients who check their results online also need less time from clinical and administrative staff. These savings more than offset the overheads of IT equipment.

Other systems have focused on the retention costs. For example, one executive's data showed an 80% reduction in the probability of a patient switching to another provider if the patient used secure messaging for consultations.

Fee for service

Efficiency and customer retention have prompted fee-for-service payments for online consultations. For example, CIGNA and Aetna are both encouraging their physicians to use the RelayHealth platform (www.relayhealth.com). CIGNA pays a physician US$25 per online consultation versus US$75 for a face-to-face one. Other payers offer up to US$35 per online consultation. CIGNA encouraged clinicians to sign up by paying for the first 3 months' fees for RelayHealth.

The UK's National Health Service is also moving in this direction. For example, the 2008 tariffs (Health Resource Groups 4) saw the introduction of a tariff for telephone-based consultations. An internet tariff is widely expected to follow.

If your payer does not cover online work, ask your manager to ask them to. A common feature of all early initiatives is that senior leaders in payers and providers agreed a framework for payments and the care that would be delivered in return. This is easier in markets with fewer players. For example, Dartmouth Hitchcock Medical Centre began its online efforts by negotiating with the three major payers in its area. The three agreed to pre-approve CPT code 99056, which covers billing for services delivered outside the physician's office at the request of the patient, and was initially designed just for alternate physical locations.

Since 2004, the American Medical Association has released new CPT codes that make negotiations much easier for all parties. Make use of these and talk to your payer.

Payments from patients

Increasingly, payers include patients. In the Arabian Gulf, early customers of Patients Know Best are adopting the platform for two reasons. First, they can attract patients from further afield. The region is geographically large, and patients are willing to travel to receive specialist care. By using our PHR software, specialists can promise to coordinate care with local providers, and minimize the need for travel, offering better service to patients.

Second, hospitals can gain revenue from mobile phone usage. Mobile phone usage is higher than in most Western markets, and customers are used to paying for premium services. Hospitals can bill for alerts about test results and mobile phone-optimized access to health care data.

The Middle East is not the only market where patients will pay. For example, Ireland's 3G Doctor offers online consultations through camera phones. These have become commonplace, as has high-speed data connectivity through 3G networks. This means that the patient can have a videophone consultation with their clinician using standard, cheap handsets. A consultation begins with the patient entering their data in the structured questionnaire of the patient portal (www.3gdoctor.com). The data are read by a physician licensed in the same region as the patient lives. After spending time researching the answer to the patient's problem, the clinician starts the videophone consultation. The most common use of the service is for patients who want a second opinion.

Second opinions can turn into full-blown relationships. For example, the University of California, San Francisco Children's Hospital, has a world-class fetal medicine team. Their website (Figure 9.1) provides valuable education content, including videos, about rare fetal conditions (http://fetus.ucsfmedicalcenter.org). This means that their site ranks highly

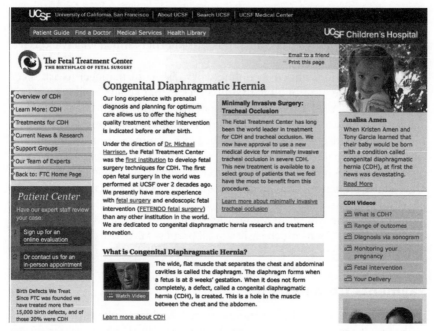

Figure 9.1 The University of California, San Francisco Children's Hospital, fetal medicine team's website.

in Google, the first place that patients turn to when confronted with diseases like congenital diaphragmatic hernia.

Once on the site, patients can click "sign up for an online evaluation." The form walks the patient through the information that the specialists need to evaluate the case, including scanned copies of ultrasound images. A multidisciplinary team of specialists reviews the case in return for US$575. And for those mothers where the recommendation is prenatal surgery, the UCSF surgeons can take over the care.

Electronic PHR workflow becomes really interesting as governments encourage patients to take over payment decisions. In the United States, health savings accounts (HSA) are tax-protected accounts that patients can spend on their care if they choose a high-deductible health plan. These have a higher threshold relative to traditional health insurance plans for the point at which the health plan takes care of payments. That means the patient is in charge of more payments earlier on.

PHRs, and working with professionals using PHRs, are likely candidates for HSA spending. The same is likely to be the case in the UK as the government is completing its trial of health budgets. This is cash, given directly to patients with chronic diseases, that they can spend on anything that contributes to their health care.

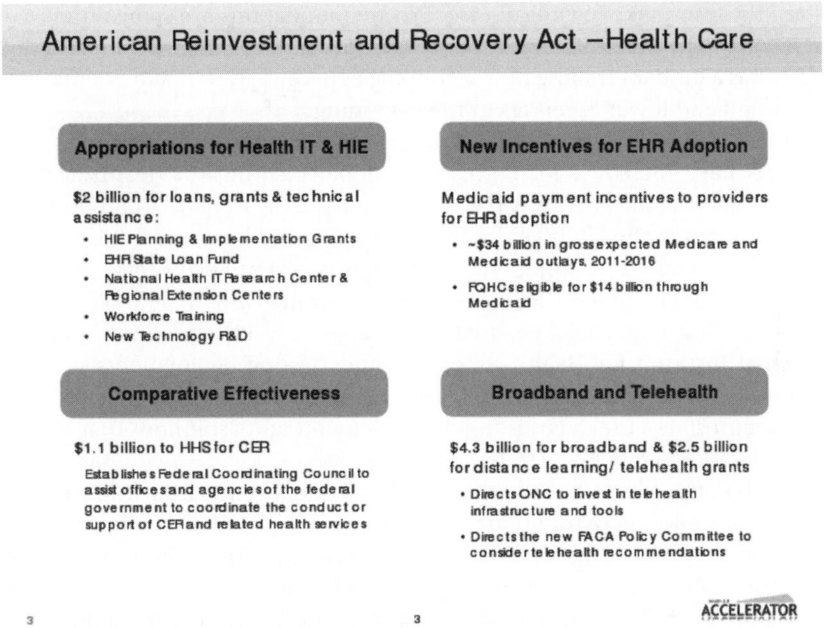

American Reinvestment and Recovery Act –Health Care

Appropriations for Health IT & HIE

$2 billion for loans, grants & technical assistance:

- HIE Planning & Implementation Grants
- EHR State Loan Fund
- National Health IT Research Center & Regional Extension Centers
- Workforce Training
- New Technology R&D

New Incentives for EHR Adoption

Medicaid payment incentives to providers for EHR adoption

- ~$34 billion in gross expected Medicare and Medicaid outlays, 2011-2016
- FQHCs eligible for $14 billion through Medicaid

Comparative Effectiveness

$1.1 billion to HHS for CER

Establishes Federal Coordinating Council to assist offices and agencies of the federal government to coordinate the conduct or support of CER and related health services

Broadband and Telehealth

$4.3 billion for broadband & $2.5 billion for distance learning/ telehealth grants

- Directs ONC to invest in telehealth infrastructure and tools
- Directs the new FACA Policy Committee to consider telehealth recommendations

ACCELERATOR

Figure 9.2 The Health 2.0 Accelerator (www.h2anetwork.org) tracks PHR companies that you can use, and the funding that they qualify for.

Capital investments

As is often the case, to earn money, you need money. Before you can benefit from the new revenue streams, you must make capital investments. Even with software as service platforms that bill you monthly based on usage, you and your team must still invest time upfront to learn how to use the system and integrate it into your existing infrastructure. The integration is from something as simple as updating your existing consent forms to integrating your patient's new software with your existing tools.

If you do not have one yet, you must get an EHR to store data that you can share with your patient's PHR. *Successfully Choosing Your EMR* (Gasch and Gasch 2010) is the sister book to this one. For US clinicians, the book covers the details of the US government's "meaningful use" criteria of the American Reinvestment and Recovery Act that qualify for funding.

For PHR investments, the Health 2.0 Accelerator (www.h2anetwork.org) is worth contacting. They track PHR companies that you can use, and the funding that they qualify for (Figure 9.2).

Research funding

But perhaps the earliest source of funding will be from research budgets. Government research agencies are interested in evaluating the contribution that PHRs can make to clinical care. Private foundations are sponsoring trials to identify best practices and develop innovations. And your own institution likely has a fund for trialing new technologies because new deployments need extra staff and lower revenues in the beginning.

In the United States, stimulus funding includes money for research, and budgets have increased for both the National Institutes of Health and the Agency for Healthcare Research and Quality. The Robert Wood Johnson Foundation has already invested heavily in personal health records research with funds phase 2 of Project Health Design (www.projecthealthdesign.org) allocated in 2009. In the UK, the Technology Strategy Board periodically provides funding that could be used to develop new PHR products, and the National Institute for Health Research funds testing deployments of PHRs within the NHS (www.nihr.ac.uk). The European Union's Eurostars program (www.eurostars-eureka.eu) is funding developments of solutions that require collaborations across EU member countries.

Collaboration tends to be important in all funding programs. Most grant evaluations allocate extra points for teams that work across institutions and across disciplines. This is why the Health 2.0 Accelerator in the United States is so useful for finding teams to collaborate with, and why we started Health-Camp UK (http://healthcamp.patientsknowbest.com) for UK collaborations.

As the technology is new, there is a lot of research. The most basic question is: do PHRs improve clinical outcomes in a double-blind randomized controlled trial? No one has done this yet, and research that gets closer to this gold standard deserves funding. Of course, double blinding is impossible when both the patient and the clinician have to be aware that they using a PHR to actually use the PHR. On the other hand, randomization is definitely possible and important as large populations of patients begin to use these tools.

Patient satisfaction scores are interesting but not important. This is because most early studies have already focused on patient satisfaction, and because it is a poor proxy. Clinical indicators such as HbA1c values for diabetics, emergency department visits from exacerbations, and average length of stay from hospitalization are all significant metrics to track. Intermediate metrics such as the time spent with each patient, and the time each patient spends, to achieve high quality are also important to demonstrate improvements in productivity.

On the other hand, best practices are important to uncover in the early stages of the research process. For example, using a new technology is almost always slower and less satisfactory in the beginning as each user is struggling to learn new habits and unlearn old ones. A study that focused on outcome metrics during the early period would likely find drops in efficiency. But if the early period is used to find the best ways of working, the rest of the study can focus on evaluating the outcomes of these ways against the older, PHR-free ones.

The risk is that we do no research. On the one hand, there was no randomized control of using the telephone, faxes, the web, or e-mail before adoption spread across all industries. Individuals and organizations just found each technology useful and so they used it more. But the PHR industry has received massive investments from large companies, and they are driving adoption before evaluation. The risk we run is adoption driven by marketing budgets rather than patient benefits, which brings us back to the real point of finding funding for this work. When this technology brings benefits to patients, it should be funded, and that in turn will expand the benefits to patients.

Summary box

- There are lots of ways to finance PHR technology.
- Ask to be paid for your work with PHRs just as all your other clinical work deserves payment.
- For salaried clinicians, institutions are integrating PHR services into their quality and efficiency efforts.
- In fee-for-service institutions, PHRs allow customer retention and offer new business models.
- In some markets, patients will pay for the increased convenience and quality of care that PHRs provide.
- Capital investments are necessary to kick-start your PHR deployment, and grants may be available for these investments.
- Research funding is also available as we explore what is possible and useful with PHRs.

References

Chen, C., Garrido, T., Chock, D., Okawa, G., and Liang, L., 2009. The Kaiser Permanente Electronic Health Record: transforming and streamlining modalities of care. *Health Affairs (Millwood)* 28(2):323–333.

Gasch, A. and Gasch, B., 2010. *Successfully Choosing Your EMR: 15 Crucial Decisions*, 1st ed. Oxford: Wiley-Blackwell.

CHAPTER 10

The future

The past had its own uncertainty, though on the whole, it wasn't as great as that of the future.

Anonymous statistician quoted by Britain's former Chancellor, Lord Norman Lamont

There will be No C, X or Q in our every-day alphabet. They will be abandoned because unnecessary. Spelling by sound will have been adopted, first by the newspapers. English will be a language of condensed words expressing condensed ideas, and will be more extensively spoken than any other.

Ladies Home Journal, December 1900, "Predictions of the Year 2000," available at http://www.yorktownhistory.org/homepages/1900_predictions.htm

The reason that you can get research funding for personal health records (PHRs) is that we are still in the early days of their technologies. As far back as 1876, Alexander Graham Bell believed that his invention, the telephone, was the best way to broadcast concerts. After successfully demonstrating this application at the Philadelphia Centennial Exposition that year, he broadcast a concert from Paris to an audience in Toronto (Sivowith 1970). Bell was relentless in finding applications for the telephone, and teaching people about these applications. For example, he installed telephones in hotels and encouraged guests to call downstairs to reception. This was how guests could understand the benefits of getting a similar system in their workplace or home (Brown and Duguid 2002).

Concerts through the phone line never caught on, however, especially as radio and then television became the mass media. Until, that is, the internet arrived as a mass medium. Most people use their phone line to access the internet. And so when Google announced its symphony orchestra competition in 2009, YouTube arguably became the best way to watch a concert without physically being in the concert hall. At www.youtube.com/symphony you can watch some of the best symphonies in the world, any time you want, along with interviews with their musicians.

Personal Health Records: A Guide for Clinicians, 1st edition. By Mohammad Al-Ubaydli.
Published 2011 by Blackwell Publishing Ltd.

PHR adopters are undergoing the same process of discovery as Bell and his contemporaries went through with the telephone. The process of learning will be faster because our generation adopts technology faster than his did, but it is still a process. And we should be prepared for surprises. I hope that you enjoy encountering these surprises as much as I do as patients and clinicians enter a new era of working together.

The future of sharing

Working in groups is hard. Doctors at Mayo faced this back in 1905 when they began adding all their paper notes to the same folder for each patient. This was the first time doctors had done this instead of keeping their own notes separate. Each of these pioneering doctors had to change their habits to suit the rest of the group, so that other doctors could read their notes rather than struggling with idiosyncracies.

The difficulties grew as other clinicians began documenting. Nurses, physiotherapists, audiologists, dieticians, and others all contribute to care. But each of them has different expertise, uses different words, and documents differently.

Patients are more different still. Do you want them writing in your medical record system?

Every clinician I talk to about PHRs is concerned that there should be one medical record rather than several. The problem, they say, with the patient having their own copy of the notes that clinicians make is that each copy would be updated differently, and the copies would have conflicting and incorrect information.

There are three possible futures, given this concern. One is that there is only one copy, and that clinicians alone are the ones that update it. This possibility is highly unlikely. Patients are using computers to make records in every aspect of their lives, from bank transactions to government documents, and health care will be no exception. If they are not allowed to update the copy that clinicians have, they will make their own copy and make changes there.

This brings us to the second possibility, one which I think the most likely: there will never be a single record. Such a record barely existed when the family physician of old maintained notes and few patients saw few specialists. But the number of copies is proliferating with the number of specialists. And more importantly, there is no other industry in which the customer and the service provider both use the same record system. Your bank does not let you edit its statement.

The customer and the service provider have different needs and workflow, and so each will work with their own copy of the data.

But an interesting future exists if the medical record becomes a wiki rather than a blog. A blog is a website that shows events in reverse chronological order, that is, with more recent events at the top of the page. Most electronic

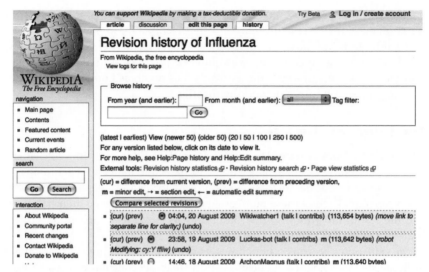

Figure 10.1 Wikis have automated version tracking.

medical record (EMR) systems today are similarly organized, showing more recent diagnoses, appointments, and prescriptions at the top.

By contrast, a wiki is a snapshot of consensus. It is a web page edited by the group and showing, at any one time, the consensus of the group. And so the record of the future may show the consensus about the patient's health. What are his or her current problems, diagnoses, treatments, and health indicators?

The magic of wikis is their automated version tracking (Figure 10.1), a technology that most clinicians and patients have not encountered. Just like the wiki encyclopedia, a wiki medical record system would constantly track who changed what, when. Every reader can be a writer, fixing errors, or revert to earlier error-free versions, as they see fit.

If wiki workflow were put to use for the medical record, the implications would be fascinating. Every member of the clinical team, including the patient, would have to be in agreement about the patient's current health.

Wikipedia is experimenting with "trust info," a tool that takes this further (Figure 10.2). For each article, the software highlights text that is not trustworthy. In Wikipedia's world, trustworthy text has been edited several times, and by users who have made trustworthy edits in the past. The software shows the peer-review process in real time. It is the most promising model to adopt if we do want a single record for the patient and clinicians.

Genomics

The contributions your patient will make to this single record will increase, and you should learn from them. Genomic medicine will probably be the specialty that most clearly turns patients from students into teachers.

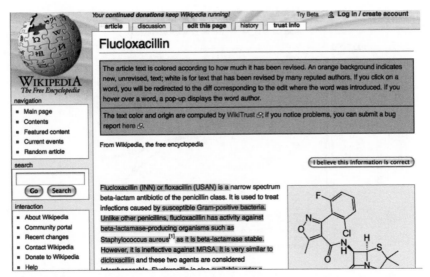

Figure 10.2 Wikipedia's trust info experiment.

This is partly because medical school curriculums have not caught up and updated their curricula to include interpreting genomic information. So when a patient comes with printout from a genomic site such as 23andMe (www.23andme.com) or Navigenics (www.navigenics.com), few clinicians are specialized enough to know how to walk the patient through the data.

But the real issue is that genomics follows the Carlson Curve (Carlson 2008), which is the rate at which the cost of sequencing drops (Figure 10.3). This rate is even faster than Moore's law (Moore 1965), which for the past 40 years has meant that computers halve in price every 18 months.

Genomic sequencing, in other words, is getting better and cheaper at a rate even faster than computers do. What costs US$1 million to sequence today would cost less than US$1,000 in 20 years. The National Human Genome Research Institute in the United States and others around the world are investing in researches that accelerate the target price of US$1,000 for sequencing a patient's complete genome.

Second, the analysis of these genes is through computers, so the rate of 1,000-fold improvements in volume and quality and quantity of analysis is also Moore's law high.

The pricing is within consumers' reach. Single condition tests are available from companies such as DNA Direct (www.dnadirect.com) for US$200–1,000. These allow a patient to test for single gene diseases like cystic fibrosis. Analysis of multiple common variations across the genome is available through single-nucleotide polymorphism companies such as Navigenics for US$2,499, DeCODEme (www.decodeme.com) for US$985, and 23andme for US$399. These provide risk assessment tests for diseases with multiple genes like rheumatoid arthritis. Whole genome scans by companies such as

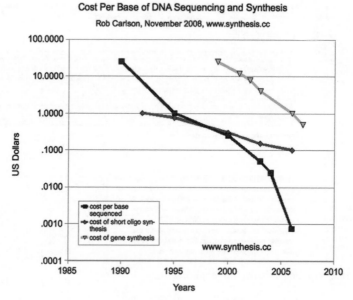

Figure 10.3 The Carlson Curve shows the rate at which the cost of sequencing drops.

Knome (www.knome.com) are available for US$99,500, down from a previous US$350,000, and are sure to drop further by the time you read this book.

Of course, sequencing is not understanding, and understanding is not acting. Consumer genomics is rising to this challenge by creating some extraordinary user interfaces. These interfaces are helpful not just to patients, but also to clinicians, as professionals' abilities to interpret statistical results are poor (Berwick et al. 1981).

The home page for a patient using 23andme, for example, shows the diseases for which the patient is at highest risk relative to the rest of the population (Figures 10.4 and 10.5). But relative risk is a concept that people find difficult to understand. So 23andme puts this in diagrams that show groups of patients (Figure 10.6) because people are better at interpreting spatial information. The website also shows the contribution of each gene to these risk scores (Figure 10.7).

Navigenics also invests in user interfaces that walk the patient through the results, and what their implications are (Figure 10.8).

So your patients will be coming to you with genetic analyses, and their explanations, faster than your medical school curriculum can ever keep up with. Continuing medical education from your professional college is not the answer: you must learn from you patient what he or she has been taught. The good news is that the genomic sequencing companies are hiring usability professionals to provide teaching resources that are both high quality and fast impact. That means that you can learn from your patient much faster than you would expect. But you must be prepared to learn.

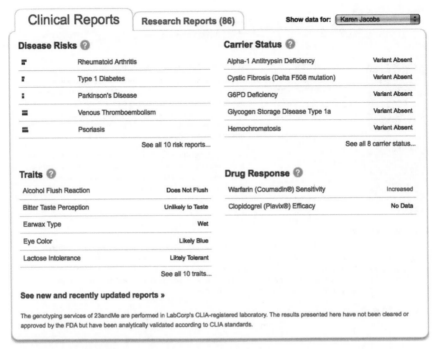

Figure 10.4 23andme shows the diseases for which the patient is at highest risk relative to the rest of the population.

Of course, that is not to say that consumer genomics is without problems. First, not all patients learn what to do with it. For example, although Navigenics includes a counseling session with each of its sequencing services, only 20% of patients take them up on this. It is unclear why the percentage is so low, but for some patients at least it seems to follow from a fatalistic interpretation of genetics. In other words, some patients believe that a genetic risk means a definite outcome, and that they cannot do anything to alter it. So

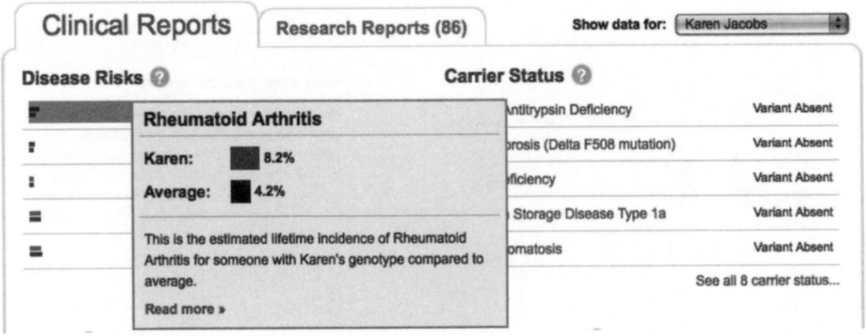

Figure 10.5 23andme shows details about the relative risk for each disease.

Your Genetic Data

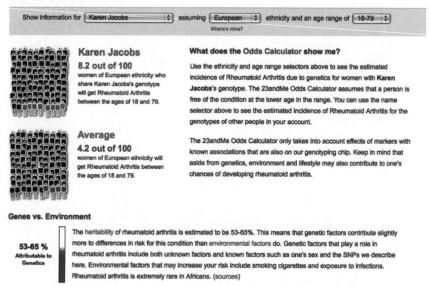

Show information for [Karen Jacobs] assuming [European] ethnicity and an age range of [18-79]
Where's mine?

Karen Jacobs

8.2 out of 100
women of European ethnicity who share Karen Jacobs's genotype will get Rheumatoid Arthritis between the ages of 18 and 79.

Average

4.2 out of 100
women of European ethnicity will get Rheumatoid Arthritis between the ages of 18 and 79.

What does the Odds Calculator show me?

Use the ethnicity and age range selectors above to see the estimated incidence of Rheumatoid Arthritis due to genetics for women with **Karen Jacobs's** genotype. The 23andMe Odds Calculator assumes that a person is free of the condition at the lower age in the range. You can use the name selector above to see the estimated incidence of Rheumatoid Arthritis for the genotypes of other people in your account.

The 23andMe Odds Calculator only takes into account effects of markers with known associations that are also on our genotyping chip. Keep in mind that aside from genetics, environment and lifestyle may also contribute to one's chances of developing rheumatoid arthritis.

Genes vs. Environment

53-65 %
Attributable to Genetics

The heritability of rheumatoid arthritis is estimated to be 53-65%. This means that genetic factors contribute slightly more to differences in risk for this condition than environmental factors do. Genetic factors that play a role in rheumatoid arthritis include both unknown factors and known factors such as one's sex and the SNPs we describe here. Environmental factors that may increase your risk include smoking cigarettes and exposure to infections. Rheumatoid arthritis is extremely rare in Africans. (sources)

Figure 10.6 23andme uses spatial diagrams to better explain relative risk.

one thing you can easily do is to encourage a patient who has paid for this service to also make use of the counselor.

More significantly, different genomic sites seem to focus on different genes, use different papers to interpret the same gene, and interpret differently from the same paper (Swan 2009). These differences are disconcerting, but on the other hand are just explicit demonstrations of the differences in opinions between different clinicians. What is likely to happen is that companies will specialize into providing either the highest quality sequencing or the highest quality analyses of the sequences. The quality of sequencing will improve through the continuous development that drives the Carlson Curve, and the quality of analysis will increase with research.

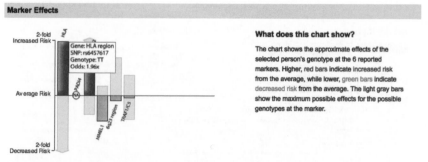

Marker Effects

2-fold Increased Risk

Gene: HLA region
SNP: rs6457617
Genotype: TT
Odds: 1.96x

Average Risk

2-fold Decreased Risk

What does this chart show?

The chart shows the approximate effects of the selected person's genotype at the 6 reported markers. Higher, red bars indicate increased risk from the average, while lower, green bars indicate decreased risk from the average. The light gray bars show the maximum possible effects for the possible genotypes at the marker.

Figure 10.7 23andme shows the contribution of each gene to relative risk scores.

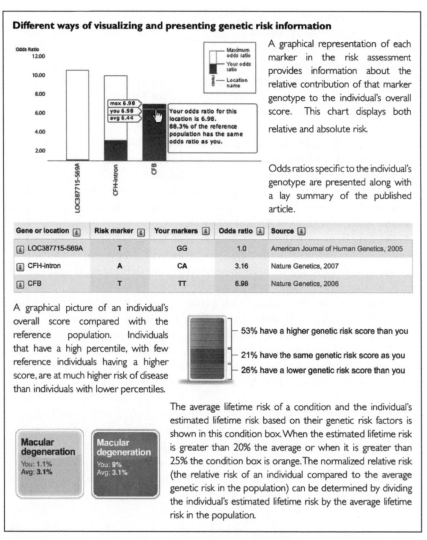

Figure 10.8 Navigenics's user interface explains genetic test results and their implications.

Using PHRs for research

Research is why Harvard Medical School started the Personal Genome Project (PGP, at www.personalgenomes.org). This offers to 100,000 individuals complete sequencing of their genomes, free of charge, as long as the participants agree to publish these sequences. Studying the patterns in the genomes of so many individuals will allow powerful conclusions, including the contribution that particular genes make to a body's response to drugs. Pretty soon, says Ryan Phelan of DNA Direct, "You would no more take a drug without knowing the relevant data from your genome than you would get a blood transfusion without knowing your blood type" (Dyson 2007).

Patients are recognizing that working online allows aggregation on a scale previously unimaginable. This scale is important for research, and that the research leads to cures.

For example, when Kathy Guisti was diagnosed with multiple myeloma back in 1996, she soon discovered that there were few promising new drugs to help her. As a businesswoman and scientist who had worked at Merck and received an MBA from Harvard, she decided to take matters into her own hand. Along with her twin sister, she founded the Multiple Myeloma Research Foundation (www.multiplemyeloma.org), which has so far raised US$160 million to support clinical research.

PHRs can help to reduce the biggest cost for this research—patient recruitment. For example, both RareShare (www.rareshare.org) and Patients-LikeMe (www.patientslikeme.com) include tools that make it easy for patients to share their data with researchers. This is not just for large-scale trials. You can use the platforms to begin small pilot studies with particular subsets of patients. Whatever you think you need, it is worth contacting the research teams at these organizations, because they do want to facilitate the most important workflow of PHRs: patients and clinicians working together to improve health care. This is not the future. The tools are already here, and I hope that this book has encouraged you to make use of them.

Thank you for reading this book, and I hope that you enjoyed it. I want to remind you that you can help me with my research for the next edition. If you do something interesting with PHRs, need to get in touch with other pioneers, or just need help with your own deployment, send me an e-mail at book@patientsknowbest.com. I look forward to hearing about your work.

Summary box

- We are in the early days of PHR technology, and have a lot to discover.
- Sharing records with patients extends the difficulties faced from sharing with other clinicians.
- The difficulties of sharing will be solved by better user interfaces, not by restricting the sharing.
- Genomics is an example area of medicine where patients will be able to learn faster than medical schools can teach doctors.
- You should learn from educated patients like these.
- PHRs provide other tools for learning that support clinical research.

References

Berwick, D.M., Fineberg, H.V., and Weinstein, M.C., 1981. When doctors meet numbers. *American Journal of Medicine* 71(6):991–998.

Brown, J. and Duguid, P., 2002. *The Social Life of Information*, 1st ed. Boston: Harvard Business Press, pp. 88.

Carlson, R., 2008. Cost per base of DNA sequencing and synthesis. [Online] (Updated November 2008) Available at: http://www.synthesis.cc/graphics/ carlson_cost_per_base_nov_08.jpg [Accessed September 7, 2009].

Dyson, E., 2007. Full disclosure. *Wall Street Journal*. 25 July 2007. Available at: http://online.wsj.com/article/SB118532736853177075.html [Accessed September 7, 2009].

Moore, G., 1965. Cramming more components onto integrated circuits. *Electronics Magazine* 38(8):4–7. Available at: ftp://download.intel.com/museum/Moores_Law/ Articles-Press_Releases/Gordon_Moore_1965_Article.pdf [Accessed August 29, 2009].

Sivowith, E., 1970. A technological survey of broadcasting's "pre-history," 1876–1920. *Journal of Broadcasting and Electronic Media*. 15(1):1–20.

Swan, M., 2009. Personal genome revolution. [Online] (Updated June 14, 2009) Available at: http://melanieswan.com/documents/Genomics_Revolution.pdf [Accessed September 7, 2009].

PART 4

Appendices

APPENDIX A

Google Health

The latest version of this guide is freely available at http://book. patientsknowbest.com, and you can share it with your patients, clinicians, colleagues, and family.

Google Health is Google's personal health record platform and is available at www.google.com/health. The Cleveland Clinic's MyChart is perhaps its most high profile user (http://mychart.clevelandclinic.org), but Beth Israel Medical Center, MinuteClinic, and other health care providers also allow patients to get a copy of their medical records through Google Health.

Google Health is designed for patients in the United States but accepts registration from outside the United States. Google's preference is for data that its computers can run calculations on. For example, you can use it to store the numbers of test results because it can plot these over time. Although you can upload a scanned piece of paper with the test results this is not quite as good because no calculations can be run on the scanned picture.

Creating an account

Registration at Google Health is free of charge at www.google.com/health (Figure A.1). Registration is only for patients, or for those who have been invited by patients to view their records. To register you need an account with Google (Figure A.2). If you have one already, for example, for your Google Mail e-mail messages (GMail), you can just sign in with your username and password and Google will create a Google Health account for you with the same details. If you do not have a Google account, you can register with any e-mail address you already have and Google will create a username for your Google Health account that is tied to your e-mail address.

Once your registration is complete, you gain access to the home page of your Google Health account. You can access this page by going to www.google.com/health and logging in with your existing or new Google account details (Figure A.3).

Personal Health Records: A Guide for Clinicians, 1st edition. By Mohammad Al-Ubaydli. Published 2011 by Blackwell Publishing Ltd.

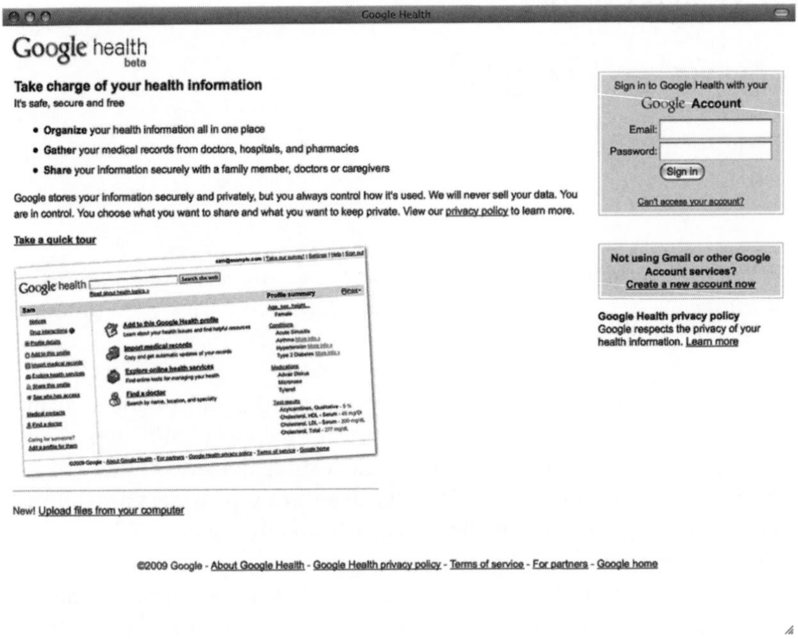

Figure A.1 Google Health at www.google.com/health.

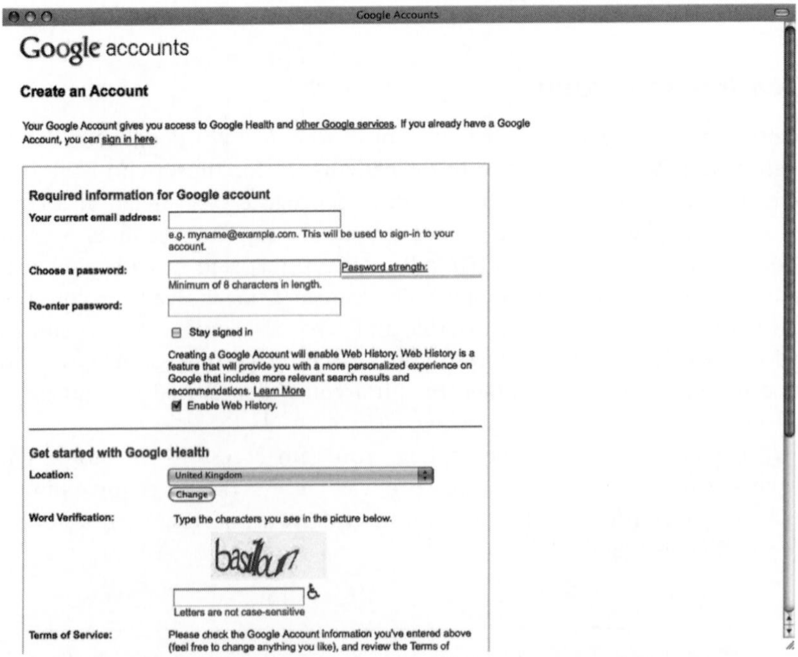

Figure A.2 Registration for Google Health requires a Google account.

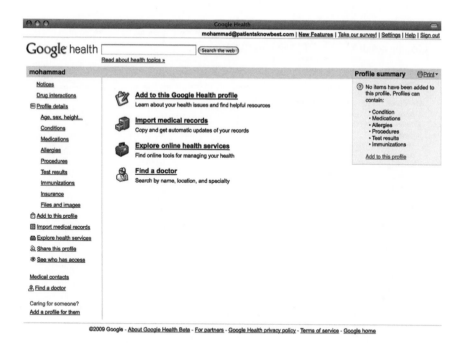

Figure A.3 The Google Health dashboard.

Adding data

There are several ways to add data. The more you automate data entry, the more likely you are to complete entry, and the less likely you will introduce errors. But automation requires effort, and sometimes money, upfront. So you should start with manual entry to experiment with the benefits. Once you know that you are finding the software useful, you can start investing in it.

To start, click on the "Add to this Google Health profile" link the top of the page (Figure A.4). By default this will take you to add to your list of conditions, for example, diabetes.

Choose from the list of diseases that Google suggests as you type in (Figure A.5). The more specific your choice, the better it is for your clinicians. For example, instead of "Diabetes," "Type 1 diabetes" tells your doctor that your diabetes is related to the immune system rather than "Type 2 diabetes," which is related to diet, or "diabetes insipidus," which is a rare and completely different illness (Figure A.6).

Click on any of the links at the top of the page to add different kinds of data. For example, for sugar results click on "Test results" and type in "Glucose."

Again, choose from the list of suggestions as you type in. For test results, you will have to add detailed numbers and units (Figure A.7).

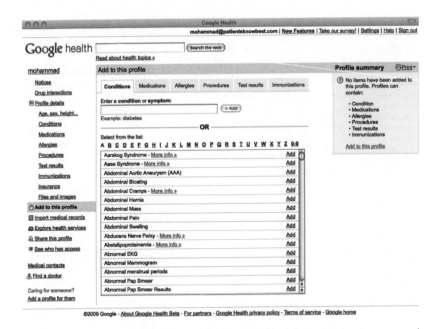

Figure A.4 You can manually add different data about your health.

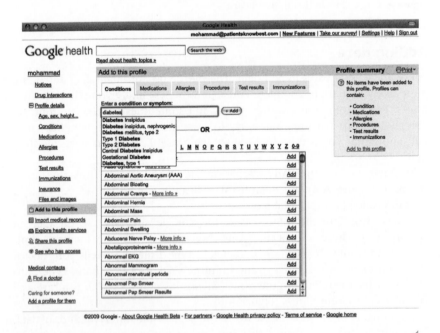

Figure A.5 Google Health suggests complete medical names when you start entering data.

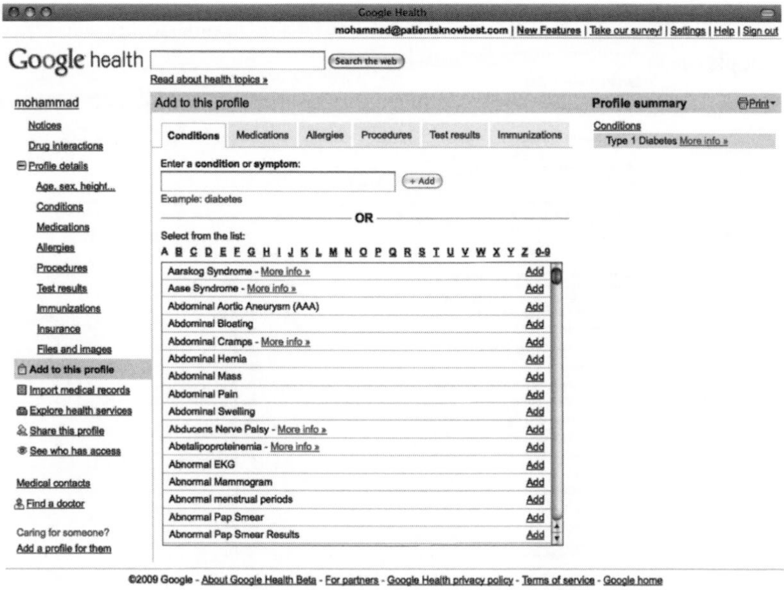

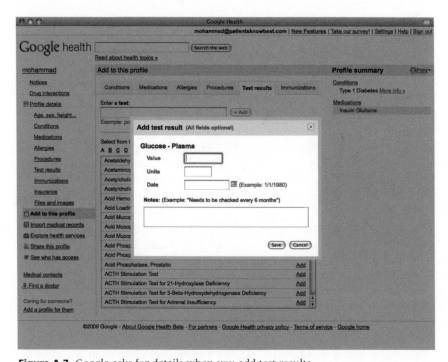

Figure A.6 Once you click on a suggestion, Google adds the item to your record.

Figure A.7 Google asks for details when you add test results.

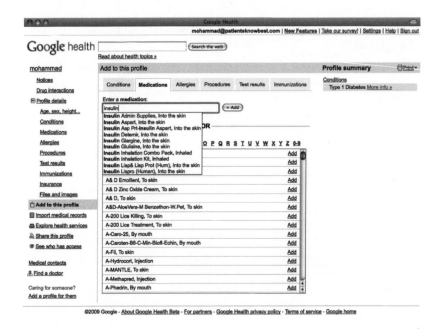

Figure A.8 Google Health also suggests complete medication names.

Include as much information as you know, and pay attention to the details. For example, units are important as they differ between different countries and have different interpretations. The "Notes" section allows details that help your clinician interpret your data and tie these to your eating habits to change your insulin dose. For example, entering "After meal" or "Before meal" is important for the sugar results of diabetics. It is helpful to also explain whether the result was high, normal, or low, as the same test result, with the same units, may mean different things in different laboratories, or even the same laboratory at different times. The piece of paper you have from the laboratory tells you the range for normal results, so you can use that to help your clinicians.

Once you have enough test results, Google can plot graphs of these results over time.

Medications also allow entering details, for example, by showing the route in which you take insulin (Figure A.8).

For all the information that you add, Google adds layers of educational materials. For example, clicking the "More info" link in conditions shows encyclopedia entries from the National Library of Medicine, while doing so in medications shows drugs information from First DataBank.

Finally, you can also upload scanned images and files. To do so, click on "Files and images" on the left-hand side (Figure A.9).

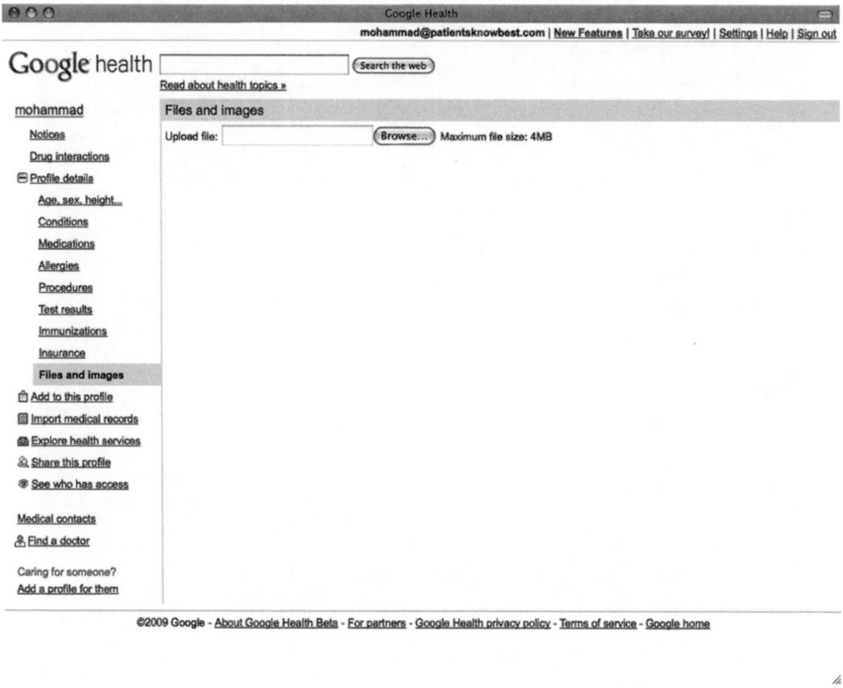

Figure A.9 You can upload scanned images and files to Google Health.

Click on the "Browse" button to find the file on your computer, and Google will copy it over to Google Health. Google cannot calculate from files, so you will not be able to plot charts or read encyclopedia entries. But having these files is better than not having any information at all as you share your records with your clinical team.

Sharing data

The "Share this profile" link at the left of the page allows you to share your records with others (Figure A.10). Click it and enter the e-mail address of the person you want to share your records with.

You need the e-mail address of this person, and Google will send them an invitation message that guides them through the technical details (Figure A.11). However, it is worth telling the person about this invitation before you send it out, or at least adding a personal message under the "Message" box.

The person you invite will be able to read everything and change nothing inside your Google Health account (Figure A.12). If in doubt, do not give

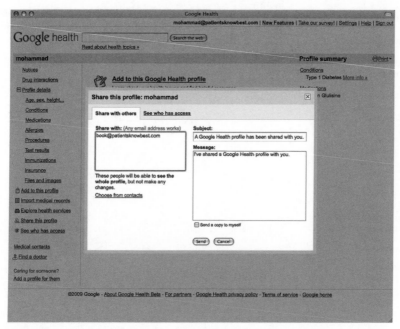

Figure A.10 The "Share this profile" link allows you to share your records with others.

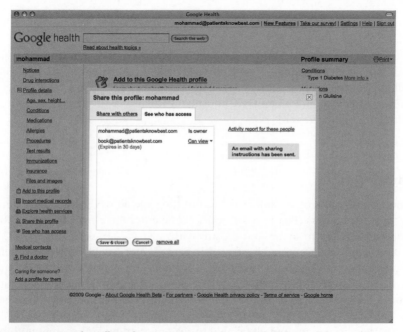

Figure A.11 Google will send an invitation to the e-mail address of the person you want to share records with.

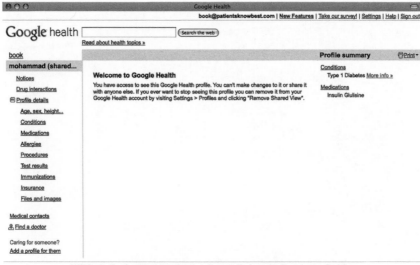

Figure A.12 The person you invite will be able to read everything and change nothing inside your Google Health account.

access. But if you know the person and they help you manage your health, you can start by giving them access knowing that you can always change your mind and revoke their access.

The person will get your message and a link to confirm their acceptance. After confirming, and if necessary, registering, the person has the same dashboard view as you do. However, on the left-hand side they can switch to viewing your account by clicking on your name.

You can also enter information on behalf of others, for example, for a relative you are caring for (Figure A.13). Under "Caring for someone?," click on "Add a profile for them" from the bottom-left corner of the page.

Enter the name of this person and click the "Save" button. The name will appear on the left-hand side of the page, close to yours. Clicking on each name allows you to enter data about the person. As you deal with more data for more of your family members, you will probably want to automate the data entry.

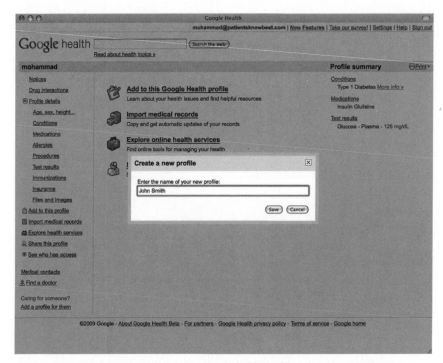

Figure A.13 You can enter information on behalf of others, for example, for a relative you are caring for.

Importing medical records

Google built Google Health so that others can build their own software on top. Such software is called "Personal health services," and you can see the list by clicking on "Import medical records" from the dashboard. Personal health services mean that you can automatically receive data from others, rather having to manually enter it yourself.

This includes getting a copy of your records from your health care providers. The importance is not just for your own access but because your own clinicians struggle to find out what other clinicians from other institutions know about you. Privacy laws and technical barriers make data sharing hard. But sharing is important to provide safe care. So the more you can store your data in one place, for your all clinicians to look at, the safer the care you can get from each clinician.

Next to each is a "Link to profile" button. To get your medications from CVS, click on the button below "CVS Caremark" (Figure A.14).

The CVS website will walk you through registration and then request authorization to send data back to your Google Health account. Make sure that you have registered at the CVS website already, or that you have the information necessary for registration. Registration for each institution requires

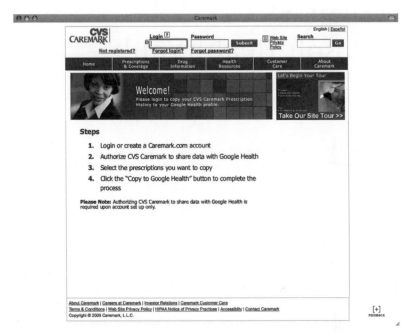

Figure A.14 To get your medications from CVS, click on the button below "CVS Caremark."

the unique number that institution has for you. For CVS it is the ExtraCare number that is on your CVS loyalty card, while for a hospital it will be your hospital ID.

Congratulations, you are now a Google Health expert. You know how to use the software to store your medical records, and those of your family members. You can share the information with the clinicians who care for you. And you can download and upload data into your records.

APPENDIX B
Microsoft HealthVault

The latest version of this guide is freely available at http://book.patients knowbest.com, and you can share it with your patients, clinicians, colleagues, and family.

HealthVault is Microsoft's personal health record platform and is available at www.healthvault.com. Some of the most prestigious health care providers to use it early on include the Mayo Clinic (http://healthmanager.mayoclinic. com) and New York Presbyterian Hospital (http://mynyp.org), and others are joining, such as the Cleveland Clinic. Patients can also download their data from pharmacies (e.g., CVS and Walgreens), upload data from medical devices, and share data with health charities and associations such as the American Cancer Society. Companies like American Well (www.americanwell.com) allow patients to store copies of the transcripts of online consultations and can view patient-entered data from a health account with patient authorization.

HealthVault is only available within certain countries. The United States was the first, of course, but Microsoft is rolling out access in other parts of the world, including Canada, the United Kingdom, and Germany in 2010. Microsoft also supports OpenID for logging in, which is a much more convenient way of tracking passwords and a progressive approach to working with other websites.

Creating an account

Registration at HealthVault is free of charge at www.healthvault.com (Figure B.1). To register as a patient, or an individual clinician to whom patients can grant access, click on "I'm an individual" (Figure B.2).

The website does a good job of explaining the platform to patients. The videos are focused on the needs of families and are worth watching. Click on "Create a free HealthVault account."

You have two options for registration (Figure B.3). You either can register with a Microsoft Windows Live ID, for example, your hotmail.com e-mail address or you can use OpenID.

Personal Health Records: A Guide for Clinicians, 1st edition. By Mohammad Al-Ubaydli. Published 2011 by Blackwell Publishing Ltd.

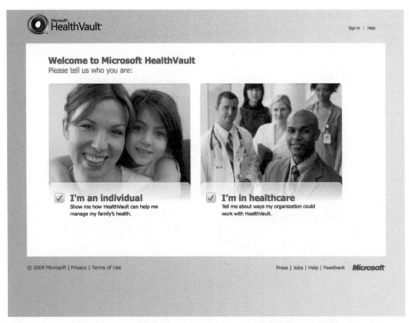

Figure B.1 Registration at HealthVault is free of charge at www.healthvault.com.

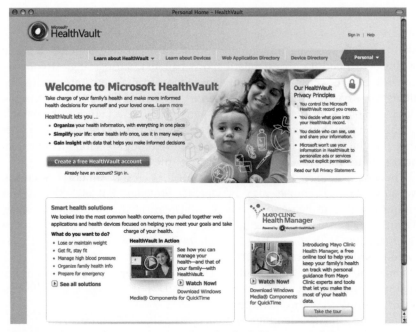

Figure B.2 Registering as a patient, or an individual clinician to whom patients can grant access.

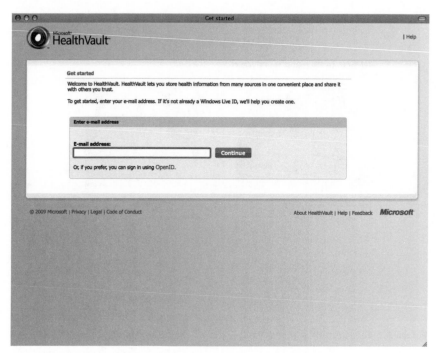

Figure B.3 You have two options for registration on HealthVault.

Microsoft is showing how progressive it is by allowing patients to log in with OpenID because this standard allows patients to use a single account to access multiple websites. Not only is this more convenient, preventing patients from having to remember different passwords for different websites, but it also prevents the normal response to this problem, which is that people choose the same password for all the websites they use. When a patient does this, they never change their password because doing so is too inconvenient across all the websites, and so the security of the password is very low.

Encourage your patients to use OpenID. Microsoft supports Microsoft Windows Live of course, also an OpenID provider, but also TrustBearer (http://openid.trustbearer.com) and MyOpenID (http://myopenid.com). TrustBearer is particularly secure because it provides a USB stick that must be used along with the password, while MyOpenID is the earliest and most widely used supporter of OpenID.

Once you have registered with an OpenID provider, you get an identifier that you can use to log in. Click on the "OpenID" link to register your Health-Vault account using this identifier.

Enter the OpenID identifier and click the "Sign in" button. The OpenID provider will ask for your password to authenticate your identity (Figure B.4), and then for permission to transfer data to HealthVault for authorization.

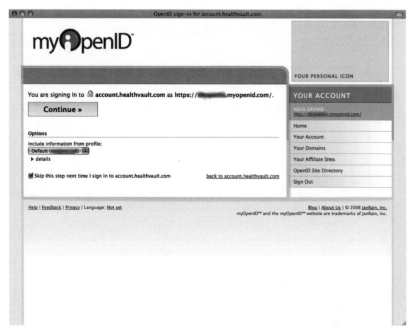

Figure B.4 The OpenID provider will ask for your password to authenticate your identity for HealthVault.

Click the "Continue" button. You will see the data transferred and can amend these data (Figure B.5). After filling out all the information, click the "Continue" button.

Once your registration is complete, you gain access to the home page of your HealthVault account (Figure B.6). In the future, you can access this page by going to www.healthvault.com and logging in with your Windows Live ID or OpenID details.

Adding data

There are several ways to add data. The more you automate data entry, the more likely you are to complete entry, and the less likely you will introduce errors. But automation requires effort, and sometimes money, upfront. So you should start with manual entry to experiment with the benefits. Once you know that you are finding the software useful, you can start investing in it.

To start, click on the "Health information" tab at the top of the page (Figure B.7). Click on any of the links on this page to add a certain kind of data. For example, for sugar results click on the plus sign to the right of "Blood glucose measurement" (Figure B.8).

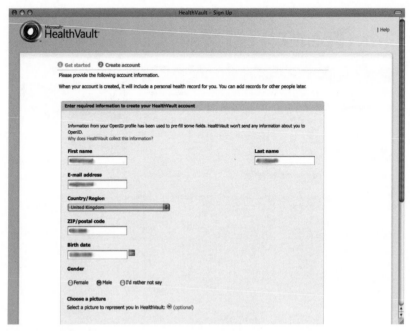

Figure B.5 OpenID transfers your data for HealthVault.

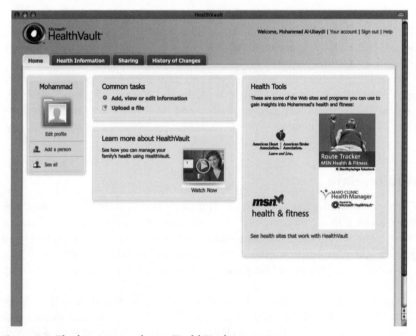

Figure B.6 The home page of your HealthVault account.

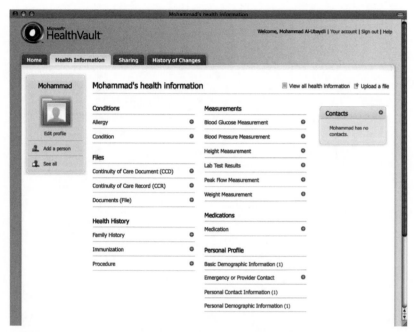

Figure B.7 To start adding data, click on the "Health information" tab.

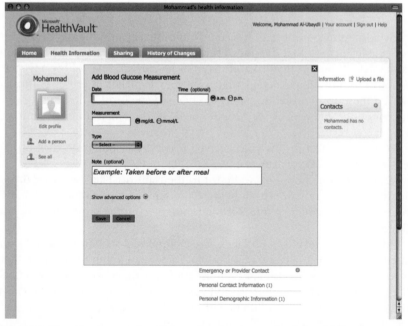

Figure B.8 To add sugar results, click on the plus sign to the right of "Blood glucose measurement."

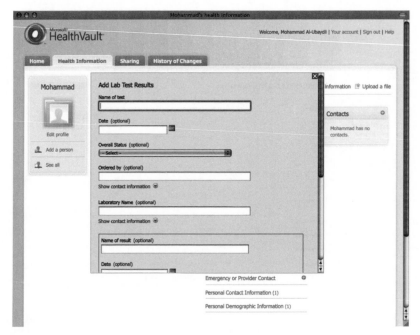

Figure B.9 To add other test results you received from your laboratory, click on the plus sign to the right of "Lab test results."

Include as much information as you know, and pay attention to the details. For example, check that the unit is the same as the one from your laboratory as the default one in HealthVault may not be correct. The "Show advanced options" section allows details that help your clinician interpret your data and tie these to your eating habits to change your insulin dose. For example, entering "After meal" or "Before meal" in the "Measurement context" list.

To add other test results you received from your laboratory, click on the plus sign to the right of "Lab test results" (Figure B.9).

Make sure you choose from the list to the right of "Flag" whether or not the result was "Normal." This is because the same value will have a different interpretation between different laboratories, or even the same laboratory on different dates.

Individual test results, with labels, are examples of structured data. Structured data are great because you can plot them on a graph or calculate their averages. However, a lot of the information you have may just be letters. These are not structured, but are still very useful for your current clinicians. You can scan these and save them within HealthVault (Figure B.10). Click on the plus sign to the right of "Documents (File)".

Click on the "Browse" button to choose your file and give it a sensible description under "Description." Be as detailed as possible, including the date

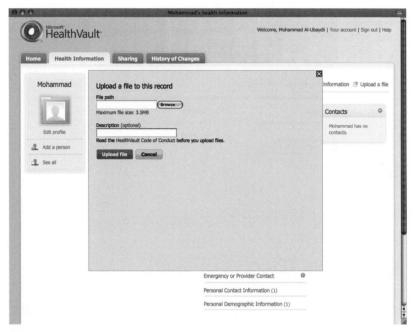

Figure B.10 You can scan printouts, faxes, or photocopies from your clinicians and save them within HealthVault.

of the letter you scanned, for example, as well as its topic, so that you and your clinician can easily find it in the future. A good description is often the only difference between unstructured data and disorganized data.

Sharing data

The "Sharing" tab at the top of the page allows you to share parts of your record with others (Figure B.11). Click on "Send a new sharing invitation" to invite a clinician, relative, or friend to look at your record (Figure B.12).

Type in the e-mail address of the person you want to share your record with. This does not have to be the e-mail address of the account that the person uses with HealthVault, but you do have to be sure that you have typed in an address that only this person can access.

There are three types of access: "View", "View and modify," and "Act as a custodian." The first two are self-explanatory, but you must be confident about the implications of the third before you grant access in this way. A custodian has the same powers you do. Not only can they view and modify the data in your health record, they can also control who else gets to do so, and even delete the entire account. If in doubt, do not give custodian access.

If you give "View" or "View and modify" access, you can choose what individual data items to give access to (Figure B.13).

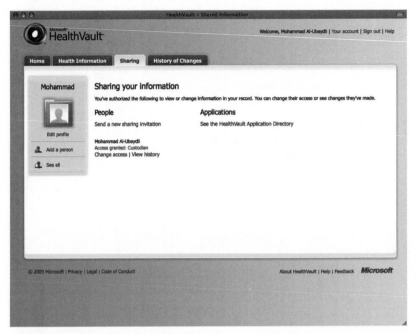

Figure B.11 The "Sharing" tab at the top of the page allows you to share parts of your record with others.

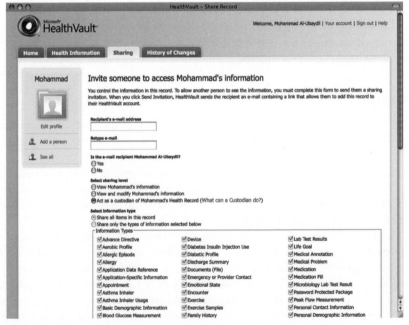

Figure B.12 Click on "Send a new sharing invitation" to invite a clinician, relative, or friend to look at your record.

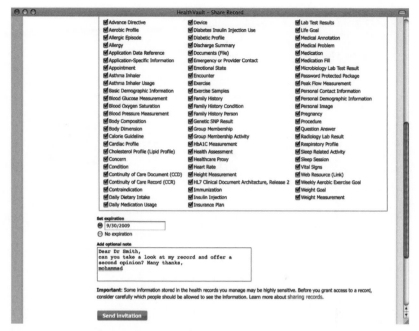

Figure B.13 You can choose which individual data items to give others access to.

Do not be fooled by the degree of control this appears to give you. For example, even if you do not allow the person you are sharing with to see your "Condition," the "Medication" may well give you away. Even accessing the "Appointment" may divulge too much information as the speciality of your clinician also suggests a narrow set of conditions from which you could be suffering.

You can set an expiration date for access, which is good for getting a one-off second opinion, or as you begin testing out the system. Finally, under "Add optional note," it is useful to enter a short, personal message reminding the clinician of who you are and when you last had an appointment. When you are ready, click the "Send invitation" button.

The person will get your message and a link to confirm their receipt and acceptance. After confirming, and if necessary, registering, the person has the same dashboard view as you do (Figure B.14). However, underneath their photo on the left-hand side, they can "Switch to" viewing your account.

Adding structured data using applications

Microsoft built HealthVault so that others can build their own software on top. This software is called a HealthVault application. Applications mean that

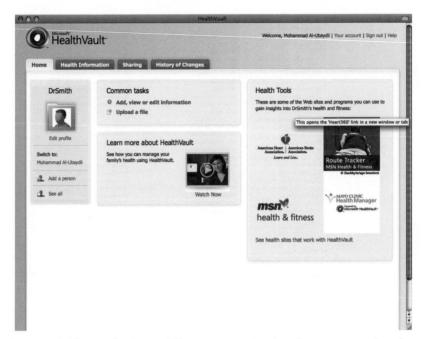

Figure B.14 After confirming, and if necessary, registering, the person you shared your records with has the same dashboard view as you do.

you can automatically receive structured data from others, rather having to manually enter it yourself.

This includes getting a copy of your records from your health care providers. This is important not just for your own access but because your own clinicians struggle to find out what other clinicians from other institutions know about you. Privacy laws and technical barriers make data sharing hard. But sharing is important to provide safe care. So the more you can store your data in one place, for your clinician to look at, the safer the care you can get from that clinician.

To start downloading your data, click on the "Sharing" tab at the top and then "See the HealthVault application directory".

Next to each is a "Try now" link. To get your medications from CVS, click on the link to the right of "My CVS/pharmacy prescriptions" (Figure B.15).

The CVS website will walk you through registration and then request authorization to send data back to your HealthVault account. Make sure that you have already registered at the CVS website, or that you have the information necessary for registration. Registration for each institution requires the unique number that institution has for you. For CVS it is the ExtraCare number that is on your CVS loyalty card, while for a hospital it will be your hospital ID.

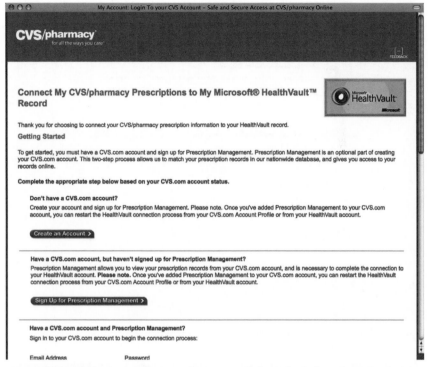

Figure B.15 To get your medications from CVS, click on the link to the right of "My CVS/pharmacy prescriptions."

If your computer is running Microsoft Windows, you can also upload data from your devices. A list of these is available at www.healthvault.com if you click on "Device directory," and it includes scales, pedometers, and glucose meters. Check that the device is compatible with HealthVault before you buy it.

Once you have it, go to www.healthvault.com/getstarted to download the software that links the device to your HealthVault account. You will need to sign into this account and then choose the people whose records you want the software to update (Figure B.16).

Click the "Continue" button. You will get a list of the data types that the device can update, for example, blood glucose and peak flow. Unlike granting other people access to your records, the access you grant here is less sensitive. It simply allows the device to add to your records rather than risking your privacy by showing these records. Each device also figures out where its data should go, so the blood glucose meter will not enter data into your peak flow diary (Figure B.17).

When you finish, click the "Allow access" button. Click on the version of Windows you are using, for example, "Vista," and the download of the

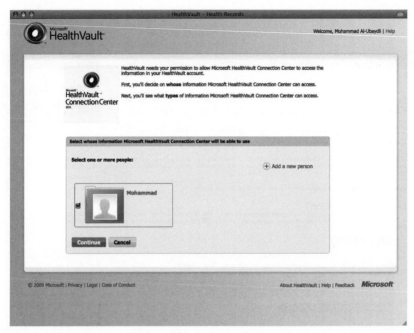

Figure B.16 If your computer is running Microsoft Windows, you can also upload data from your devices.

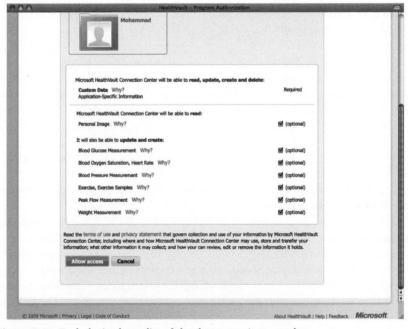

Figure B.17 Each device has a list of the data types it can update.

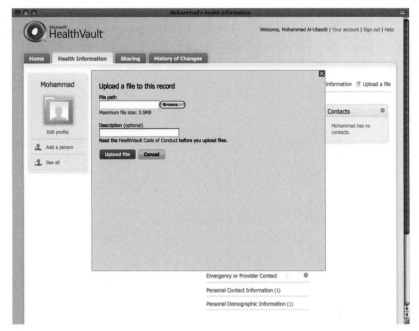

Figure B.18 HealthVault can import CCR files.

installation software will begin. Once complete, start the installer and follow its instructions. Once the installation is complete, you can run Health-
Vault connection center at any point from the "Start" menu. Make sure
you have it running before your connect your new device and then select
the device from the list below "What type of device do you want to use?"
The software will walk you through the installation and integration with
HealthVault.

Finally, it is worth understanding the abbreviation CCR as it will be increasingly helpful in the future. The continuity of care record is a format for storing
medical data just as DOC is a format for storing Microsoft Word documents.
Personal health record software companies, including Microsoft and Google,
use the CCR standard to exchange data with health care providers and with
medical devices. So if you want someone to manually give you a copy of your
record before their institution has integrated with Microsoft HealthVault, ask
that they give you the copy in CCR format.

HealthVault can import CCR files in the "Health information" tab. Click on
the plus sign to the right of "Continuity of care record (CCR)" (Figure B.18).

Click on the "Browse" button to choose the file. Under "Description" enter the date on which the file was created for you, the name of the institution that provided you with the file, and the contents of the file. Click
the "Upload file" button, and the new structured data appear inside your
record.

Congratulations, you are now a HealthVault expert. You know how to use the software to store your medical records, and those of your family members. You can share the information with the clinicians who care for you, and you can download and upload data into your records.

Index

Abbreviations, use of, 34
American Recovery and Reinvestment
    Act of 2009, 65
Association of Cancer Online Resources,
    23

Blog, 75

Capital investments, 71
Carlson Curve, 77, 78
Cisco devices, 49
Clinical teams and PHRs, 30–38
    benefit to whole team, 31–2
    learning from patients, 36
    reaction to errors, 34–6
    readable writing, 33–4
    relationship with patients, 33
    relatives help, use of, 36–8
    training for team
        changes to workflow, 33
        importance of PHRs, 32
        use of software, 33
Clinician-led PHRs, 58
Community Health Network, 67
Confidentiality, maintenance of, 34
Consent forms, 40
Continua data standard, 59
Continuity of care document (CCD)
    format, 57
Continuity of care record (CCR) format,
    57, 59
Custom search engine site, creation of,
    41–2

Data formats, PHR, 57
Data Protection Act, European Union,
    64, 65
Department of Veterans Affairs, 37, 67
Doctors.net, UK, 17

Educational resources, identification of,
    41–3

Education, for patients, 39–45
    data gathering, importance of, 42, 44
    encouragement, need of, 39
    identification of useful resources, 41–3
    informing consent, 40–41
EHR vendors, 58
Electronic health records (EHRs),
    xvii–xviii, 58
Eurostars program, EU, 72

Facebook, 17
Face-to-face appointment, need of, 46–7
Federal Trade Commission (FTC), 65
Finance, 67–73
    capital investments, 71
    fee for service, 68–9
    payment for working online, request
        for, 67
    payments from patients, 69–70
    research funding, 71–3
    salaried clinicians, 67–8
Finding the Right EHR, xviiii, 58

Genetic Information Nondiscrimination
    Act (GINA), 15
Genomics, 76–81
Google, 20
Google custom search engine, 41–2
Google Health, 59, 87
    adding data on, 89–93
    creating account on, 87, 88
    dashboard, 87, 89
    importing medical records, 96–7
    registration for, 87, 88
    sharing data on, 93–6

Hannan, Dr. Amir, 3
Health 2.0 Accelerator, 71, 72
HealthCamp UK, 72
Health information exchange (HIE),
    60

Health Insurance Portability and
    Accountability Act (HIPAA), 64–5
Health savings accounts (HSA), US, 70
HealthVault. *See* Microsoft HealthVault
HealthVault application, 107–8

Information technology (IT), 55–62
  building blocks in
    data, 55
    hardware, 55
    networks, 56
    software, 56
  data collection from patients, 59
  and outsourcing options, 60–62
  and PHR data, 56–7
  PHR hardware, 57–8
  PHR software, 58–9
  regional data networks, 60
Informing consent, 40–41
  background reading, 40
  competency testing, 40
Internet, power of, 20
IT department, outsourcing of, 60–62
iWantGreatCare, 25

Journal of Participatory Medicine, xiii

Kaiser Permanente, 67, 68

Laws
  for building trust between doctor and
      patient, 62
  EU Data Protection Act, 63
  ownership of data by patients, 62
  patients responsibilities, 65–6
  in United States, 64–5

MD Anderson Cancer Center, 4–5
MedHelp, 25
Medscape, 6
Microsoft HealthVault, 59, 98–112
  adding data on, 101, 103–5
  adding structured data by applications,
      107–111
  creating account on
    free of charge registration, 98, 99
    OpenID, use of, 100–102
    options for registration, 98, 100

sharing data on, 105–8
  users of, 98
Moderator Community, 25
Multiple Myeloma Research Foundation,
    82

National Institutes of Health (NIH), 20
  Patient-Reported Outcomes
      Measurement Information
      System, 10
Nature, 20
Navigenics, 77, 81
NHS Evidence website, UK, 6

Omron Healthcare, 59
Online consultations, 49–50
Online delivery of information, 50–51
Online discussions, importance of, 23–4
OpenNotes Project, 6

Paper diaries, 7
Participatory medicine movement,
    xiii–xiv. *See also* Patient
    communities
Patient Access Electronic Records System
    (PAERS), xix
Patient communities, 19–26
  communicating in, 25–6
  value of, 23–4
  Wikipedia, 20–23
Patient-led PHR deployments, 58
Patient Opinion, 25, 26
Patient portal, xviiii–xix
  VUMC, 4
PatientsLikeMe, 7–8, 13, 16, 39, 82
Personal Genome Project (PGP), 81–2
Personal health record (PHR), xv, xvii,
    xix–xx
  for clinical research, 81–2
  emergencies and, 44–5
  finance for (*See* Finance)
  future of sharing of, 75–7
  laws and (*See* Laws)
  paper *vs.* electronic, xix–xx, xvii
  technology of, benefits of (*See* Clinical
      teams and PHRs)
Personal health services, 96
Phones, as PHR hardware, 57
phpBB, software, 25

Privacy, protection of, 13–18
  advice to patients on, 15–16
  of professionals, 17–18
  from relatives, 14–15
  security of PHR, ensuring of, 14
Project HealthDesign, 11
Protected health information (PHI),
    63–4

Regional data networks, 60
Regional Health Information
    Organizations (RHIOs), US, 60
RelayHealth platform, 68
ReliefInsite, 8–9
Research funding, 71–3
Robert Wood Johnson Foundation, 6,
    11, 72
Rorschach test, 6–7

Security, of patient's records, 14
Sermo, United States, 17
Sharing data, 3–12
  for building trust, 3
  data from patients, 7–9
  data not in traditional health records,
    collection of, 9–11
  early access, benefits of, 6
  and learning by patients, 6–7
  risks of, lowering of, 4
  for safety, 4
  sharing control and ownership in,
    11–12
Shipman, Dr.Harold, 3
Successfully Choosing Your EMR, 71

3G Doctor, xix, 33, 69
Time saving, with PHR, 46–51
  face-to-face appointment, need of,
    46–7
  online consultations, 49–50
  online delivery of information, 50–51

sharing benefits with patients, 48–9
team members on, discussion with,
    47–8
telephone consultations, 47
"Trust info" tool, Wikipedia, 76, 77
23andMe, 77–80

Vanderbilt University Medical Center
    (VUMC), 4

Web-based patient-led PHR software, 58
Websites
  Cisco's care-at-a-distance solutions, 49
  Continua data standard, 59
  DNA Direct, 77
  Google Health, 87
  Health 2.0 Accelerator, 71
  HealthVault, 98
  Hello Health, xix
  Moderator Community, 25
  NHS Evidence website, 6
  Omron Healthcare, 59
  OpenNotes Project, 6
  PAERS, xix
  participatory medicine movement, xiii
  PatientsLikeMe, 7–8, 82
  phpBB, 25
  RareShare, 36, 82
  ReliefInsite, 8
  Rorschach test, 6
  3G Doctor, xix, 33
  University of California, San Francisco
    Children's Hospital, 69–70
  ZumeLife, 9, 10
Wiki, 75–6
Wikipedia, 20–23
  fixing errors in, 20–23
Wikipedians, 20
Writing, patient-friendly, 33–4

ZumeLife, 9